STOMACH ULCER DIET COOKBOOK FOR BEGINNERS

99+ Delicious and Nutrient-Rich Anti-Inflammatory Recipes to Aid in Stomach Healing and Reverse Ulcers.

Kingsley Klopp

Copyright © 2024 All rights reserved.

No part of this book may be reproduced or transmitted in any form or by any means, electronic or mechanical, including photocopying, recording, or by any information storage and retrieval system, without written permission from the author. The scanning, uploading, and distribution of this book via the internet or via any other means without the permission of the author is illegal and punishable by law. The author has made every effort to ensure the accuracy of the information contained in this book. However, the author cannot be held responsible for any errors or omissions.

Table of Contents

Introduction..7

Part 1
Understanding Stomach Ulcers.
- What Are Stomach Ulcers?...9
- Causes and Risk Factors...11
- Symptoms and Diagnosis..14
- The Role of Diet in Managing Stomach Ulcers......................17
- Foods to Avoid..19
- Foods to Include...22

Breakfast Recipes
Oatmeal Porridge..24
Banana Yogurt Smoothie...25
Boiled Sweet Potatoes..26
Cottage Cheese with Melon..27
Mashed Potatoes...28
Pumpkin Porridge...29
Vegetable Omelet..30
Smoothie Bowl..31
Polenta..32
Carrot and Ginger Juice...33
Squash Soup..34
Steamed Vegetables..35
Quinoa Salad...36
Sweet Potato Hash..37
Cauliflower Toast..38
Almond Rice Porridge..39
Soft Boiled Eggs..40
Barley Soup..41
Omelet with Herbs...42
Zucchini Bread..43
Millet Porridge..44
Pear Smoothie...45
Buckwheat Pancakes..46
Rye Bread Sandwich..47
Basil and Spinach Smoothie...48

Poultry Recipes

Chicken and Carrot Noodles...49
Turkey and Oat Porridge...50
Chicken Cauliflower Fried Rice..51
Baked Turkey and Eggplant...52
Chicken and Avocado Salad..53
Turkey and Potato Soup..54
Steam-Fried Chicken Drumsticks..55
Turkey Vegetable Loaf..56
Slow Cooked Chicken with Oats...57
Herbed Turkey Steaks..58
Chicken Paillard..59
Turkey Spinach Meatloaf..60
Chicken and Parsnip Stew..61
Stuffed Chicken Breast...62
Turkey and Carrot Patties...63
Chicken and Peas Pilaf...64
Chicken and Potato Bake...65
Turkey Quinoa Salad..66
Baked Chicken and Mushrooms..67
Turkey and Squash Skillet..68
Chicken Porridge..69
Chicken and Zucchini Boats...70
Turkey and Sweet Potato Hash..71
Oat-Crusted Turkey Cutlets..72
Chicken and Vegetable Stir-fry...73
Turkey Meatballs...74

Fish & Seafood Recipes

Steamed Cod..75
Poached Salmon...76
Baked Tilapia..77
Grilled Shrimp...78
Clam Soup..79
Baked Haddock..80
Ginger Shrimp Stir Fry..81
Oven-Poached Flounder..82
Salmon and Potato Bake..83
Shrimp and Rice Pilaf...84
Crab Stuffed Mushrooms...85
Scallops with Peas..86
Mackerel in Oatmeal..87

Lobster and Rice..88
Salmon Salad...89
Grilled Sole..90
Clam and Potato Casserole...91
Baked Sea Bass...92
Poached Pear and Salmon..93
Scallop Soup...94
Halibut and Zucchini..95
Cod and Asparagus Bake..96
Tilapia with Minted Peas..97
Crab and Spinach Noodles...98
Scallops with Parsnip Puree...99

Vegetables
Vegetable Stew...100
Pumpkin and Carrot Bake..101
Herbed Potato Salad..102
Spinach and Ricotta Stuffed Shells..103
Mushroom and Barley Soup..104
Oven-Roasted Kohlrabi..105
Cream of Mushroom Soup...106
Vegetable Quinoa Pilaf..107
Fennel and Carrot Slaw...108
Sweet Pea and Potato Puree...109
Green Bean Almondine...110
Stuffed Zucchini...111
Leek and Potato Soup...112
Butternut Squash Risotto..113
Roasted Parsnips...114
Carrot and Coriander Soup...115
Celery Root Mash..116
Steamed Brussels Sprouts...117
Stewed Green Beans...118

Desserts
Carrot Cake...119
Mango Mousse..120
Vanilla and Honey Panna Cotta..121
Banana Ice Cream...122
Warm Apple Cider...123
Oatmeal Smoothie..124

10-WEEK MEAL PLAN..125

To show our appreciation for your purchase, we're delighted to offer you these special bonuses as a heartfelt thank you.

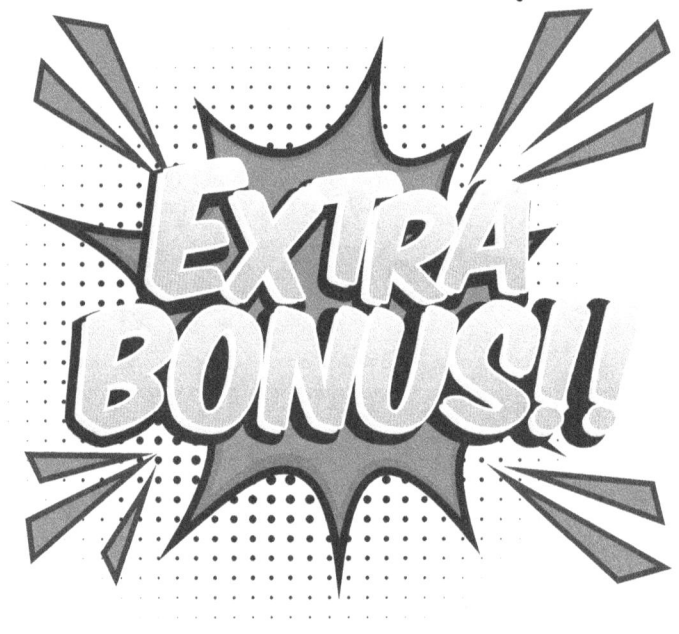

1. A Food Tracker Journal
2. Downloadable E-BOOK featuring full-color images of finished recipes

Important Note

We understand that everyone's body is different, and individual dietary needs can vary, Your body is unique, and what works for one person may not work for another. While the recipes in this cookbook are crafted to be gentle on the stomach and promote healing, it's essential to listen to your body. If a particular ingredient doesn't agree with you or if you have specific dietary restrictions, feel empowered to make adjustments as needed. Your health and comfort come first.

Consulting with your healthcare provider is also crucial, especially if you have any concerns or uncertainties about how to integrate these recipes into your diet. Your doctor knows your medical history best and can provide personalized guidance to ensure that the foods you choose align with your overall treatment plan.

Please note that the nutritional information provided with each recipe is approximate. Actual values may vary based on factors such as ingredient brands, portion sizes, and cooking methods. We encourage you to use this information as a general guideline and to consider consulting with a nutritionist for precise dietary advice tailored to your needs.

Furthermore, If our cookbook has brought joy to your kitchen and table, we'd be thrilled to hear about your experiences in an Amazon review. On the flip side, if you stumble upon any hiccups while exploring our recipes, don't hesitate to get in touch at **kloppkingsley@gmail.com.** We're here to support your cooking journey every step of the way.

Introduction.

Imagine waking up every day to a gnawing pain in your stomach, a constant reminder that your diet isn't just about taste—it's about survival. Stomach ulcers can turn each meal into a challenge, making you question every bite. But what if there was a way to transform your meals into something that not only nourishes you but also soothes and heals your body? Welcome to the **Stomach Ulcer Diet Cookbook for Beginners,** where you'll find the tools and recipes to make eating enjoyable again.

Living with a stomach ulcer can be daunting, and the mere thought of eating can bring anxiety. The pain, the discomfort, and the fear of aggravating your condition can overshadow the joy that food should bring. But it doesn't have to be that way. This cookbook is here to guide you through the dietary maze, providing you with delicious, ulcer-friendly recipes that are both satisfying and beneficial for your stomach health. Picture this: you're in your kitchen, surrounded by fresh ingredients, the aroma of herbs and spices filling the air. Cooking is not just about preparing food; it's about creating a space of healing and comfort. This book is your companion in that journey, offering you simple, flavorful recipes that cater specifically to your needs. We understand that a stomach ulcer doesn't just impact what you eat, but also how you live. That's why this cookbook isn't just a collection of recipes—it's a guide to reclaiming your life through food.

Let's talk about what makes this cookbook unique. Each recipe is carefully crafted with ingredients that are gentle on your stomach while still packing a punch in the flavor department. We believe that eating for health doesn't mean sacrificing taste. Whether it's a soothing soup, a comforting main dish, or a refreshing smoothie, every recipe is designed to be both delicious and easy to prepare, even for beginners. You don't need to be a gourmet chef to make these meals; all you need is a willingness to experiment and a desire to nurture your body. Stomach ulcers require special attention when it comes to diet, but that doesn't mean your meals have to be bland or boring. In this cookbook, we emphasize foods that are low in acidity and rich in nutrients, helping to heal your gut and reduce irritation. Think of creamy oatmeal topped with bananas and honey, or grilled chicken with a side of steamed vegetables—all bursting with flavor and designed to be kind to your stomach. Each recipe comes with tips on how to adapt it to your tastes and needs, ensuring that you have the flexibility to make each meal your own.

But this book is about more than just recipes. It's about understanding your condition and learning how to manage it through diet. We provide insights into the best foods to include in your diet, as well as those to avoid, empowering you to make informed choices that support your healing journey. Armed with this knowledge, you'll feel more in control of your condition, and less like it's controlling you. We also understand that everyone's experience with stomach ulcers is different. What works for one person might not work for another, and that's okay. This cookbook encourages you to listen to your body, experiment with different recipes, and find what works best for you. It's all about trial and error, and we're here to support you every step of the way. You're not alone in this journey, and with a little patience and creativity, you can rediscover the joy of eating.

As you turn the pages of this cookbook, we hope you'll find not just recipes, but also inspiration and encouragement. Eating with a stomach ulcer can be challenging, but it's also an opportunity to reconnect with your body and learn what truly nourishes it. Every meal is a step towards healing, and we're excited to be a part of that journey with you. So, roll up your sleeves, grab your apron, and let's get cooking. Together, we'll explore a world of flavors that won't just satisfy your taste buds, but also promote a healthier, happier stomach. Welcome to a new chapter of delicious healing.

Part 1

Understanding Stomach Ulcers.

What Are Stomach Ulcers?

Stomach ulcers, also known as peptic ulcers, are painful sores that develop on the lining of the stomach, small intestine, or esophagus. They occur when the thick layer of mucus that protects the stomach from digestive acids is reduced, allowing the acids to erode the tissues lining the stomach. This condition has afflicted humans for centuries, casting a shadow over the lives of those who endure its discomfort and pain.

A Historical Perspective

The history of stomach ulcers dates back to ancient times, with descriptions of symptoms resembling those of ulcers found in ancient Egyptian, Greek, and Roman medical texts. The renowned Greek physician Hippocrates, often regarded as the father of medicine, documented cases of individuals suffering from severe abdominal pain, a hallmark of stomach ulcers. However, the understanding of this condition was rudimentary, and treatments were largely based on trial and error.

In the Middle Ages, the condition continued to be shrouded in mystery. Physicians of that era, influenced by humoral theory, believed that ulcers were caused by an imbalance of bodily fluids. Treatments included a variety of herbal concoctions, bloodletting, and dietary restrictions. The effectiveness of these treatments was questionable, and many patients continued to suffer in silence. The Renaissance period brought a renewed interest in the human body and its ailments. Anatomists began to dissect human cadavers, leading to a more accurate understanding of the digestive system. However, the exact cause of stomach ulcers remained elusive. It wasn't until the late 19th and early 20th centuries that significant strides were made in the field of gastroenterology.

Scientific Breakthroughs and Evolution of Understanding

In the early 20th century, physicians began to explore the role of stomach acid in ulcer formation. The discovery of hydrochloric acid in the stomach and its corrosive potential led to the hypothesis that excessive acid production could be a primary cause of ulcers. This marked a turning point in the understanding of the condition, leading to the development of antacids and acid-reducing medications. The most significant breakthrough came in the 1980s when Australian researchers Dr. Barry Marshall and Dr. Robin Warren identified a bacterium called Helicobacter pylori (H. pylori) as a major culprit in the development of stomach ulcers. Their groundbreaking research challenged the prevailing belief that stress and lifestyle were the primary causes of ulcers. Initially met with skepticism, their findings were eventually validated, earning them the Nobel Prize in Physiology or Medicine in 2005.

The discovery of H. pylori revolutionized the treatment of stomach ulcers. It shifted the focus from merely managing symptoms to addressing the root cause. Antibiotic therapy, combined with acid-suppressing medications, became the cornerstone of ulcer treatment, leading to significant improvements in patient outcomes. This paradigm shift not only provided relief to millions of sufferers but also underscored the importance of scientific inquiry and perseverance in advancing medical knowledge.

The Human Experience of Stomach Ulcers
Living with a stomach ulcer can be an incredibly challenging experience, marked by persistent discomfort and a constant battle to manage symptoms. The pain, often described as a burning or gnawing sensation in the abdomen, can disrupt daily activities, robbing individuals of their peace of mind. This pain is typically exacerbated by meals, creating a distressing cycle where eating, an essential and often enjoyable part of life, becomes a source of dread.

For many, the journey with stomach ulcers begins with a sense of bewilderment. The initial symptoms might be dismissed as mere indigestion or attributed to stress. As the condition progresses, the pain intensifies, prompting a visit to the doctor. The diagnosis can come as a relief, providing a name and explanation for the suffering, but it also ushers in a new set of challenges. Adapting to dietary restrictions, remembering to take medications, and navigating the social implications of having a chronic condition all add layers of complexity to daily life.

Emotions run high in this journey. The initial relief of diagnosis can quickly give way to frustration and anxiety. Questions abound: "Why me?" "What did I do wrong?" The answers are often complex and multifaceted, intertwining genetic predispositions, bacterial infections, and lifestyle factors. Support from loved ones and healthcare professionals becomes crucial, offering both practical assistance and emotional comfort.

The Modern Approach to Managing Stomach Ulcers
Today, the approach to managing stomach ulcers is comprehensive and multifaceted. It involves not only medical treatment but also lifestyle modifications. Patients are encouraged to avoid foods and beverages that can irritate the stomach lining, such as spicy foods, alcohol, and caffeine. Smoking cessation is strongly advised, as smoking can exacerbate the condition and hinder the healing process.

The medical community continues to explore new avenues for treatment and prevention. Research into the microbiome, the collection of microorganisms living in our digestive tracts, holds promise for understanding how to maintain a healthy balance of bacteria and prevent infections like H. pylori. Advances in medical technology, such as endoscopy, allow for early detection and more precise treatment of ulcers.

Causes and Risk Factors of Stomach Ulcers

Causes of Stomach Ulcers
1. **Helicobacter pylori Infection:**
   - One of the most common causes of stomach ulcers is infection with the bacterium Helicobacter pylori (H. pylori). This bacterium disrupts the mucous layer that protects the stomach lining from acidic digestive juices, leading to inflammation and ulcer formation. The exact mechanism by which H. pylori causes ulcers is complex and involves the bacteria's ability to produce enzymes and toxins that weaken the mucosal defenses and provoke an inflammatory response.
2. **Nonsteroidal Anti-Inflammatory Drugs (NSAIDs):**
   - Regular use of NSAIDs, such as aspirin, ibuprofen, and naproxen, is another major cause of stomach ulcers. These medications inhibit the production of prostaglandins, which are substances that help maintain the protective lining of the stomach. Without sufficient prostaglandins, the stomach becomes more susceptible to damage from stomach acids.
3. **Excessive Stomach Acid Production:**
   - Conditions that increase the production of stomach acid, such as Zollinger-Ellison syndrome, can also lead to the development of ulcers. This rare condition involves tumors in the pancreas or duodenum that cause the stomach to produce excessive amounts of acid, overwhelming the mucosal defenses.
4. **Other Causes:**
   - Other factors, such as radiation therapy and certain viral infections, can also contribute to the development of stomach ulcers, although these are less common.

Risk Factors for Stomach Ulcers
1. **Lifestyle Factors:**
   - Smoking: Smoking is a significant risk factor for stomach ulcers. It not only increases the likelihood of developing an ulcer but also impairs the healing process of existing ulcers. Smoking increases stomach acid production and reduces the production of bicarbonate, which neutralizes acid, thereby damaging the stomach lining.
   - Alcohol Consumption: Excessive alcohol intake can irritate and erode the mucous lining of the stomach, leading to inflammation and bleeding. It also increases stomach acid production, which further exacerbates the risk of ulcer development.
   - Diet: While diet alone is not a direct cause of stomach ulcers, certain foods and beverages can aggravate symptoms and hinder the healing process. Spicy foods, acidic foods (like citrus fruits and tomatoes), and caffeinated beverages can irritate the stomach lining.

2. Psychological Factors:
- Stress: Although stress alone does not cause stomach ulcers, it can exacerbate existing conditions and contribute to the onset of symptoms. Chronic stress can lead to behaviors like smoking and increased alcohol consumption, which are known risk factors. Stress also stimulates the production of stomach acid, which can compromise the stomach lining.

3. Genetic Factors:
- A family history of stomach ulcers can increase an individual's risk, suggesting a genetic predisposition to conditions that lead to ulcers. This could involve inherited traits that affect the stomach's ability to produce protective mucus or control acid production.

4. Medical Conditions:
- Certain medical conditions, such as liver disease, kidney disease, and chronic obstructive pulmonary disease (COPD), are associated with a higher risk of developing stomach ulcers. These conditions may alter blood flow or the immune response, making the stomach lining more vulnerable to damage.

5. Age:
- The risk of developing stomach ulcers increases with age. Older adults are more likely to be taking NSAIDs for chronic pain and other conditions, which raises their risk. Additionally, the production of protective mucus decreases with age, making the stomach lining more susceptible to acid damage.

6. Use of Certain Medications:
- In addition to NSAIDs, other medications such as corticosteroids, anticoagulants, selective serotonin reuptake inhibitors (SSRIs), and bisphosphonates can increase the risk of stomach ulcers. These medications can either directly irritate the stomach lining or exacerbate the effects of other risk factors.

7. Dietary Habits and Irregular Eating Patterns:
- Skipping meals or having irregular eating patterns can lead to increased acid production, which may damage the stomach lining. Eating large meals, particularly those high in fat, can also increase the risk of ulcers by delaying stomach emptying and increasing acid exposure.

8. Helicobacter pylori Transmission:
- The transmission of H. pylori is not fully understood but is believed to occur through contaminated food, water, or close contact with an infected person. Living in crowded or unsanitary conditions increases the risk of acquiring this bacterium.

Comprehensive Management and Prevention

Understanding the causes and risk factors of stomach ulcers is fundamental for both prevention and effective treatment. Key preventive measures include:

- Avoiding excessive use of NSAIDs: Using alternative pain relievers when possible, such as acetaminophen, which does not damage the stomach lining.
- Eradicating H. pylori infection: If diagnosed, appropriate antibiotic therapy should be pursued to eliminate the infection.
- Modifying lifestyle habits: Quitting smoking, reducing alcohol consumption, managing stress, and maintaining a healthy diet can significantly reduce the risk of developing ulcers.
- Regular medical check-ups: For those with a family history or other risk factors, regular monitoring and early intervention can help prevent complications.

Symptoms and Diagnosis of Stomach Ulcers

Symptoms of Stomach Ulcers
The symptoms of stomach ulcers can vary widely among individuals, but there are some common signs that often indicate the presence of an ulcer:

1. **Abdominal Pain:**
   - The most common symptom of a stomach ulcer is a burning or gnawing pain in the upper abdomen, usually between the breastbone and the navel. This pain can be sharp or dull and often occurs when the stomach is empty, such as between meals or during the night. It can temporarily subside after eating or taking antacids but tends to return.
2. **Nausea and Vomiting:**
   - Ulcers can cause nausea, which may be mild or severe. In some cases, vomiting occurs, which can sometimes include blood (hematemesis) or material that looks like coffee grounds, indicating bleeding in the stomach.
3. **Bloating and Belching:**
   - Individuals with stomach ulcers may experience bloating, a feeling of fullness, or increased belching. These symptoms can be uncomfortable and interfere with daily activities.
4. **Loss of Appetite and Weight Loss:**
   - Due to the pain and discomfort associated with eating, people with stomach ulcers may lose their appetite, leading to unintentional weight loss.
5. **Heartburn or Acid Reflux:**
   - Some people with stomach ulcers experience heartburn or acid reflux, which is a burning sensation that rises from the stomach to the chest.
6. **Fatigue:**
   - Chronic ulcers can lead to slow, internal bleeding, resulting in anemia. This condition can cause fatigue, weakness, and pale skin.
7. **Bloody or Dark Stools:**
   - Blood in the stool, which can appear as black or tarry stools (melena), is a sign of bleeding from an ulcer and requires immediate medical attention.
8. **Back Pain:**
   - In some cases, the pain from a stomach ulcer can radiate to the back.

Diagnosis of Stomach Ulcers

Diagnosing a stomach ulcer involves a combination of a patient's medical history, physical examination, and various diagnostic tests. Here are the key steps in the diagnostic process:

1. **Medical History and Physical Examination:**
   - The diagnostic process begins with a thorough medical history and physical examination. The doctor will ask about the patient's symptoms, their duration, and any factors that alleviate or worsen them. The physician will also inquire about the patient's use of medications, particularly NSAIDs, and any history of smoking or alcohol consumption.
2. **Laboratory Tests:**
   - Blood tests may be conducted to check for anemia, which can result from chronic blood loss due to an ulcer. Additionally, tests for Helicobacter pylori (H. pylori) infection, a common cause of ulcers, can be performed. These tests include blood antibody tests, stool antigen tests, and urea breath tests.
3. **Endoscopy (Esophagogastroduodenoscopy or EGD):**
   - An endoscopy is a key diagnostic tool for identifying stomach ulcers. During this procedure, a thin, flexible tube with a camera (endoscope) is inserted through the mouth and into the stomach and duodenum. This allows the doctor to directly visualize the ulcer and assess its size and location. The procedure also enables the physician to take tissue samples (biopsies) for further examination, particularly to test for H. pylori or to rule out cancer.
4. **Upper Gastrointestinal (GI) Series:**
   - An upper GI series, also known as a barium swallow, is an X-ray examination of the upper digestive system. The patient drinks a barium solution, which coats the lining of the stomach and small intestine, making them visible on X-ray images. This test can help identify ulcers and other abnormalities in the digestive tract.
5. **H. pylori Testing:**
   - Besides blood tests, specific tests for detecting H. pylori include:
     - Urea Breath Test: The patient drinks a special liquid containing urea. If H. pylori is present, it will break down the urea, releasing carbon dioxide, which is then detected in the patient's breath.
     - Stool Antigen Test: This test detects H. pylori antigens in a stool sample.
     - Endoscopic Biopsy: During an endoscopy, a biopsy sample can be taken and tested for H. pylori.
6. **Additional Imaging Tests:**
   - In some cases, additional imaging tests such as a CT scan or MRI may be required to assess complications of ulcers, such as perforation or obstruction.

Complications Requiring Immediate Attention

While many ulcers can be managed with medication and lifestyle changes, some complications require immediate medical attention:

1. **Bleeding:**
   - Bleeding from a stomach ulcer can be life-threatening. Symptoms include vomiting blood, black or tarry stools, and severe weakness or dizziness.
2. **Perforation:**
   - An ulcer can create a hole in the wall of the stomach or small intestine, leading to peritonitis, a severe abdominal infection. This condition causes sudden, intense abdominal pain and requires emergency surgery.
3. **Obstruction:**
   - Ulcers can cause swelling and scarring that blocks the passage of food through the digestive tract, leading to vomiting and weight loss. This condition often requires surgical intervention.

The Role of Diet in Managing Stomach Ulcers

The Healing Power of Food

The relationship between diet and stomach ulcers is profound and multifaceted. The food we eat directly interacts with the stomach lining, influencing the production of stomach acid, the integrity of the mucous barrier, and the overall health of the digestive system. For individuals with stomach ulcers, making thoughtful dietary choices can significantly reduce symptoms and promote healing.

1. **Gentle on the Stomach:**
   - Foods that are gentle on the stomach play a crucial role in ulcer management. These include bland, non-acidic, and easily digestible foods that do not irritate the stomach lining. Examples include:
     - Bananas: These fruits are not only easy to digest but also help neutralize stomach acid.
     - Oatmeal: A soothing breakfast option that provides fiber without causing irritation.
     - Boiled or steamed vegetables: Such as carrots, broccoli, and spinach, which are nutrient-rich and gentle on the stomach.
     - Lean proteins: Including chicken, turkey, and fish, which provide essential nutrients without excessive fat content that can increase stomach acid production.

2. **Hydration and Healing:**
   - Staying well-hydrated is vital for overall health and particularly beneficial for individuals with stomach ulcers. Water helps maintain the mucous barrier that protects the stomach lining and dilutes stomach acid. Herbal teas, especially those containing chamomile or ginger, can also be soothing. Chamomile has anti-inflammatory properties, while ginger aids digestion and reduces nausea.

3. **Avoiding Irritants:**
   - Equally important as incorporating soothing foods is the need to avoid irritants that can exacerbate ulcer symptoms. These include:
     - Spicy foods: Such as hot peppers and curries, which can irritate the stomach lining.
     - Acidic foods and beverages: Including citrus fruits, tomatoes, and caffeinated drinks, which increase stomach acid and cause discomfort.
     - Alcohol: Known to erode the stomach lining and increase acid production.
     - Caffeine: Found in coffee, tea, and certain sodas, which can stimulate stomach acid secretion.

Emotional and Psychological Impact

The journey of managing stomach ulcers through diet is not just about physical health; it also touches the emotional and psychological realms. Food is a source of comfort, joy, and social connection. Adapting to a new diet can feel restrictive and isolating, especially when it involves giving up favorite foods or altering long-standing eating habits. However, it's important to focus on the positive impact these changes can have on overall well-being and quality of life.

1. **Empowerment through Knowledge:**
   - Learning about which foods help and which harm can be empowering. Knowledge is a powerful tool that can turn a seemingly uncontrollable situation into one where individuals have a say in their own healing process. Understanding the reasons behind dietary recommendations can foster a sense of purpose and control.
2. **Finding Joy in New Foods:**
   - Embracing a new diet doesn't mean sacrificing enjoyment. It can be an opportunity to discover new foods and flavors that are both delicious and healing. Experimenting with different recipes, such as a soothing oatmeal topped with bananas and honey or a flavorful chicken and vegetable stir-fry, can bring back the joy of eating.
3. **Support and Community:**
   - Sharing the journey with others can make a significant difference. Support groups, both online and in-person, offer a platform to exchange tips, recipes, and encouragement. Knowing that others are navigating similar challenges can provide comfort and camaraderie.

Long-Term Strategies for Ulcer Management

Dietary changes are a crucial part of a comprehensive strategy to manage stomach ulcers. However, they should be complemented by other lifestyle modifications and medical treatments for optimal results.

1. **Regular Meals:**
   - Eating smaller, more frequent meals can help regulate stomach acid production and prevent the stomach from becoming too full, which can cause discomfort.
2. **Stress Management:**
   - Stress is a known trigger for ulcer flare-ups. Incorporating stress-reducing practices such as yoga, meditation, or even simple deep-breathing exercises can have a positive impact on digestive health.
3. **Medical Adherence:**
   - Following prescribed treatments, including medications to reduce stomach acid and antibiotics to treat H. pylori infection, is essential. Dietary changes work best in conjunction with medical treatments.

Foods to Avoid

Spicy Foods
Spicy foods are notorious for irritating the stomach lining, which can aggravate ulcer symptoms. The capsaicin in hot peppers and other spicy ingredients can increase stomach acid production and lead to a burning sensation, making symptoms worse. Common spicy foods to avoid include:
- Hot peppers (such as jalapeños, habaneros, and chili peppers)
- Spicy sauces (like hot sauce, sriracha, and chili paste)
- Spicy seasonings (such as cayenne pepper and chili powder)

Acidic Foods and Beverages
Acidic foods can exacerbate ulcer pain by increasing stomach acid levels and irritating the stomach lining. It is important to avoid foods and drinks with high acidity, such as:
- Citrus fruits (like oranges, lemons, limes, and grapefruits)
- Tomatoes and tomato-based products (such as tomato sauce, ketchup, and salsa)
- Vinegar and vinegar-based condiments (including pickles and salad dressings)
- Carbonated beverages (soda, sparkling water, and other fizzy drinks)

Caffeinated Drinks
Caffeine stimulates stomach acid production, which can worsen ulcer symptoms and delay healing. It is best to limit or avoid:
- Coffee (both regular and decaffeinated, as decaf still contains some caffeine and acids)
- Tea (especially black and green tea, which contain caffeine)
- Energy drinks
- Certain sodas (particularly colas, which contain caffeine and acids)

Alcohol
Alcohol is a significant irritant to the stomach lining. It can increase acid production, disrupt the mucous barrier, and delay the healing of existing ulcers. Individuals with stomach ulcers should avoid:
- Beer
- Wine
- Spirits (such as vodka, whiskey, rum, and gin)
- Cocktails (often containing acidic mixers like citrus juices and soda)

Fatty and Fried Foods
High-fat and fried foods can be difficult to digest and may increase stomach acid secretion. They can also slow down the emptying of the stomach, leading to increased discomfort. Foods to avoid include:
- Fried foods (like fried chicken, French fries, and fried fish)
- Fast food (such as burgers, fried snacks, and pizza)
- High-fat meats (like bacon, sausage, and fatty cuts of beef or pork)
- Full-fat dairy products (including whole milk, cheese, and butter)

Chocolate
Chocolate contains both caffeine and a compound called theobromine, which can increase stomach acid production and cause discomfort. It's best to avoid all forms of chocolate, including:
- Dark chocolate
- Milk chocolate
- White chocolate
- Chocolate-flavored desserts (such as chocolate cake, cookies, and ice cream)

High-Salt Foods
Excessive salt intake can irritate the stomach lining and exacerbate ulcer symptoms. Foods high in salt to avoid include:
- Processed meats (such as deli meats, hot dogs, and canned meats)
- Packaged snacks (like chips, pretzels, and salted nuts)
- Canned soups and vegetables (which often contain high levels of added salt)
- Pre-packaged meals and frozen dinners

Dairy Products
While not all dairy products need to be avoided, some people find that full-fat dairy products can worsen their symptoms. It's best to limit or avoid:
- Whole milk and cream
- Full-fat cheese
- Butter
- Rich, creamy desserts (like custard, ice cream, and cheesecake)

Certain Vegetables
Although vegetables are generally good for health, some can cause increased gas and bloating, which may exacerbate ulcer pain. These include:
- Onions
- Garlic
- Bell peppers
- Raw cruciferous vegetables (such as broccoli, cauliflower, and cabbage)

Processed and Refined Foods

Processed and refined foods often contain additives, preservatives, and artificial ingredients that can irritate the stomach lining. Foods to avoid include:
- Packaged baked goods (such as cookies, cakes, and pastries)
- Refined grains (like white bread, white rice, and regular pasta)
- Sugary cereals
- Pre-packaged snack foods

Mint and Peppermint

While mint is often soothing for many digestive issues, it can actually relax the lower esophageal sphincter, leading to increased acid reflux and discomfort for ulcer sufferers. Avoid:
- Peppermint tea
- Mint-flavored candies and gums
- Mint extracts used in cooking and baking

Managing a diet when you have a stomach ulcer involves making thoughtful choices to avoid foods that can exacerbate symptoms and hinder healing. By steering clear of spicy, acidic, caffeinated, alcoholic, fatty, salty, and processed foods, individuals can significantly reduce their discomfort and promote a more conducive environment for healing. Additionally, paying attention to individual triggers and maintaining a balanced, soothing diet can make living with a stomach ulcer more manageable and improve overall quality of life.

It's important to remember that each person's experience with stomach ulcers can vary, and dietary tolerances are highly individual. Consulting with a healthcare provider or a registered dietitian can provide personalized guidance and help create a diet plan that supports healing and minimizes discomfort. In the journey of managing stomach ulcers, diet becomes not just a necessity but a powerful ally in achieving better health and well-being.

Foods to Include

Healing and Soothing Foods

1. Fruits (Non-Acidic and Low-Fiber):
   - Fruits that are non-acidic and low in fiber are gentle on the stomach and can be easily digested. These fruits can provide essential vitamins and minerals without irritating the stomach lining.
     - Bananas: Known for their natural antacid properties, bananas can help neutralize stomach acid and provide a soothing effect.
     - Apples (without the skin): Peeled apples are less acidic and easier to digest, offering a good source of fiber and antioxidants.
     - Melons: Watermelon, cantaloupe, and honeydew are low-acid fruits that are hydrating and gentle on the stomach.
     - Papaya: Contains papain, an enzyme that aids digestion and soothes the stomach.

2. **Vegetables:**
   - Vegetables are packed with essential nutrients and can be prepared in ways that are easy on the stomach.
     - Leafy greens: Such as spinach and kale, which are rich in vitamins A, C, and K.
     - Carrots: Can be steamed or boiled to reduce fiber content, making them easier to digest.
     - Sweet potatoes: Baked or boiled, they are nutritious and gentle on the stomach.
     - Zucchini: Soft and easy to digest when cooked.

3. **Whole Grains:**
   - Whole grains provide fiber and nutrients without causing excessive acid production or irritation.
     - Oatmeal: A soothing and easy-to-digest breakfast option that helps reduce stomach acid.
     - Brown rice: A gentle grain that provides essential nutrients and is easier to digest than white rice.
     - Quinoa: A protein-rich grain that is gentle on the stomach and versatile in meals.

4. **Lean Proteins:**
   - Protein is essential for healing, but it's important to choose lean sources that do not exacerbate symptoms.
     - Chicken and turkey: Skinless and prepared without heavy seasoning, these proteins are easy to digest.
     - Fish: Such as salmon and cod, which are rich in omega-3 fatty acids that can reduce inflammation.
     - Eggs: Soft-boiled or poached, eggs provide a gentle source of protein.

5. **Dairy Products (Low-Fat or Non-Fat):**
    - While full-fat dairy can be irritating, low-fat or non-fat options can be included in a stomach ulcer-friendly diet.
        - Low-fat yogurt: Contains probiotics that promote gut health and aid digestion.
        - Skim or low-fat milk: Provides calcium without the added fat that can irritate the stomach.
        - Low-fat cheese: Such as cottage cheese, which is easy to digest and nutritious.
6. **Healthy Fats:**
    - Incorporating healthy fats into the diet can support overall health without irritating the stomach.
        - Olive oil: A healthy fat that can be used in cooking and dressings.
        - Avocado: Rich in healthy fats and gentle on the stomach when eaten in moderation.
        - Nuts and seeds: Such as almonds and chia seeds, which provide healthy fats and nutrients. These should be consumed in small quantities to avoid irritation.
7. **Herbs and Spices:**
    - Mild herbs and spices can add flavor without causing irritation.
        - Ginger: Known for its anti-inflammatory and digestive benefits.
        - Turmeric: Contains curcumin, which has anti-inflammatory properties.
        - Chamomile: Often used in tea form, it can soothe the digestive system.
8. **Beverages:**
    - Staying hydrated is crucial, and certain beverages can help soothe the stomach.
        - Herbal teas: Such as chamomile, ginger, and licorice tea, which can reduce inflammation and promote healing.
        - Aloe vera juice: Known for its soothing properties, it can help heal the stomach lining.
        - Water: Essential for overall health and digestion, aim to drink plenty of water throughout the day.

Breakfast Recipes

1. Oatmeal Porridge
Ingredients
- 1 cup rolled oats
- 2 cups water
- 1 cup low-fat milk or almond milk
- 1 banana, sliced
- 1 tablespoon honey
- 1 teaspoon ground cinnamon
- 1/4 teaspoon ground nutmeg
- 1/4 cup blueberries (optional)

Instructions
1. In a medium-sized pot, bring the water to a boil.
2. Add the rolled oats and reduce the heat to a simmer. Cook for 5 minutes, stirring occasionally.
3. Stir in the milk and continue to cook for another 5 minutes, or until the oats are soft and the porridge reaches your desired consistency.
4. Remove the pot from the heat and stir in the honey, ground cinnamon, and ground nutmeg.
5. Serve the oatmeal porridge in bowls, topped with sliced banana and blueberries if desired.

Nutrition Info (per serving)
- Calories: 220
- Protein: 6g
- Carbohydrates: 40g
- Fiber: 6g
- Sugars: 14g
- Fat: 3g
- Saturated Fat: 1g
- Sodium: 50mg

Serves
- 2 servings

Cooking Time
- **Total time: 15 minutes**

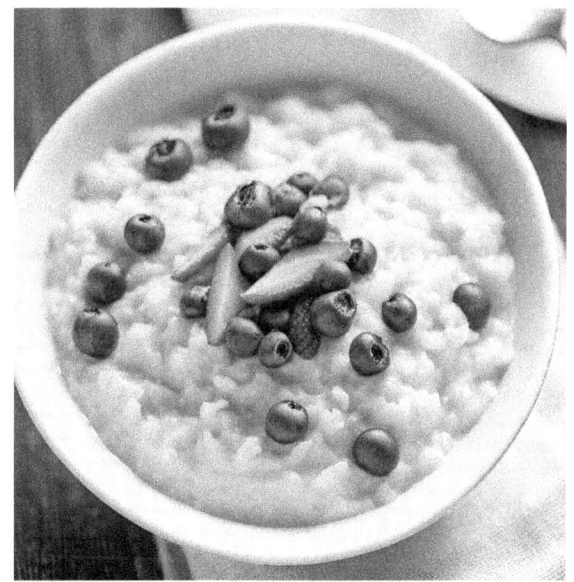

2. Banana Yogurt Smoothie

Ingredients
- 1 ripe banana
- 1 cup low-fat yogurt (plain or vanilla)
- 1/2 cup almond milk
- 1 tablespoon honey
- 1 teaspoon ground flaxseed
- 1/2 teaspoon vanilla extract
- 4-5 ice cubes

Instructions
1. In a blender, combine the banana, low-fat yogurt, almond milk, honey, ground flaxseed, vanilla extract, and ice cubes.
2. Blend on high until smooth and creamy.
3. Pour the smoothie into a glass and serve immediately.

Nutrition Info (per serving)
- Calories: 180
- Protein: 7g
- Carbohydrates: 34g
- Fiber: 3g
- Sugars: 25g
- Fat: 3g
- Saturated Fat: 1g
- Sodium: 75mg

Serves
- 1 serving

Cooking Time
- **Total time: 5 minutes**

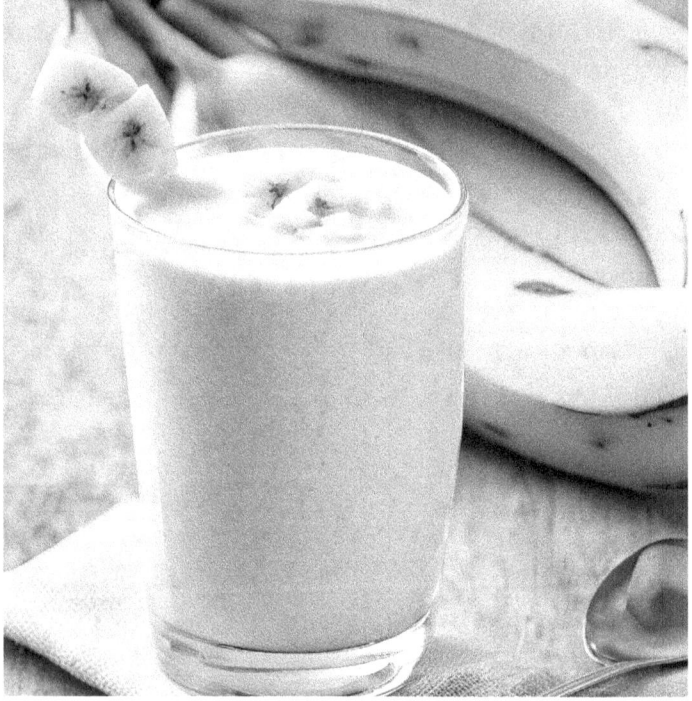

3. Boiled Sweet Potatoes

Ingredients
- 2 medium sweet potatoes
- 1 tablespoon olive oil
- 1 teaspoon ground cinnamon
- 1 tablespoon honey

Instructions
1. Peel the sweet potatoes and cut them into 1-inch cubes.
2. Place the sweet potato cubes in a large pot and cover them with water.
3. Bring the water to a boil, then reduce the heat to a simmer. Cook the sweet potatoes for 15-20 minutes, or until they are tender when pierced with a fork.
4. Drain the sweet potatoes and return them to the pot.
5. Add the olive oil, ground cinnamon, and honey. Mash the sweet potatoes until smooth and well combined.
6. Serve warm.

Nutrition Info (per serving)
- Calories: 160
- Protein: 2g
- Carbohydrates: 35g
- Fiber: 5g
- Sugars: 12g
- Fat: 3g
- Saturated Fat: 0.5g
- Sodium: 40mg

Serves
- 2 servings

Cooking Time
- **Total time: 30 minutes**

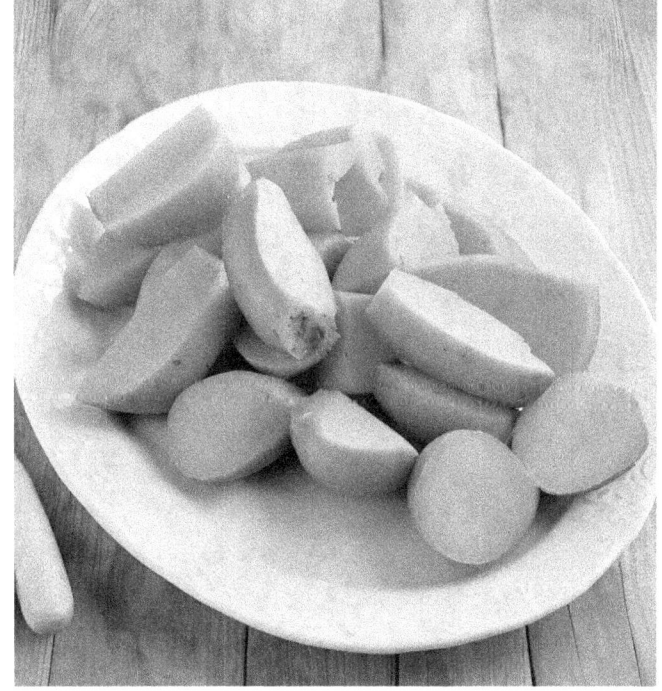

4. Cottage Cheese with Melon

Ingredients

- 1 cup low-fat cottage cheese
- 1 cup melon (cantaloupe or honeydew), cubed
- 1 tablespoon honey
- 1/2 teaspoon ground cinnamon

Instructions

1. In a bowl, combine the cottage cheese and cubed melon.
2. Drizzle the honey over the top.
3. Sprinkle with ground cinnamon.
4. Serve immediately.

Nutrition Info (per serving)

- Calories: 180
- Protein: 14g
- Carbohydrates: 24g
- Fiber: 2g
- Sugars: 22g
- Fat: 4g
- Saturated Fat: 1.5g
- Sodium: 340mg

Serves

- 1 serving

Cooking Time

- Total time: 5 minutes

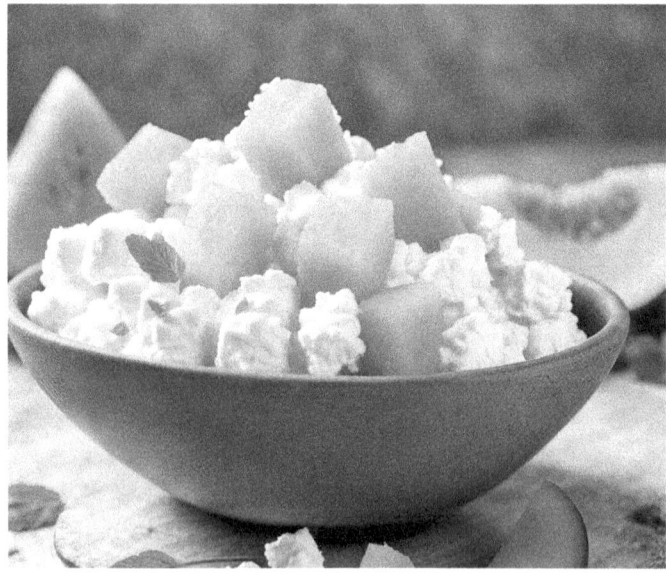

5. Mashed Potatoes

Ingredients
- 2 large potatoes, peeled and cubed
- 1/4 cup low-fat milk
- 1 tablespoon unsalted butter
- 1 teaspoon ground nutmeg

Instructions
1. Place the peeled and cubed potatoes in a large pot and cover with water.
2. Bring the water to a boil, then reduce the heat to a simmer. Cook the potatoes for 15-20 minutes, or until tender.
3. Drain the potatoes and return them to the pot.
4. Add the low-fat milk and unsalted butter.
5. Mash the potatoes until smooth.
6. Sprinkle with ground nutmeg and stir to combine.
7. Serve warm.

Nutrition Info (per serving)
- Calories: 140
- Protein: 3g
- Carbohydrates: 25g
- Fiber: 3g
- Sugars: 2g
- Fat: 4g
- Saturated Fat: 2.5g
- Sodium: 20mg

Serves
- **2 servings**

Cooking Time
- **Total time: 30 minutes**

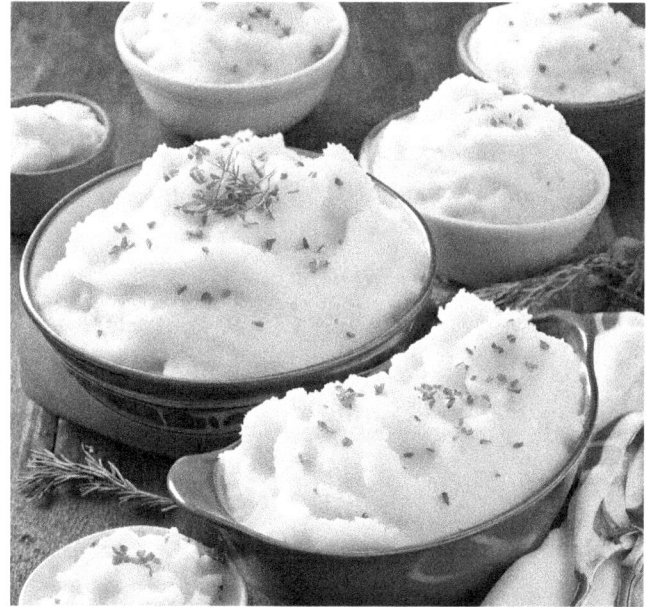

6. Pumpkin Porridge

Ingredients
- 1 cup pumpkin puree (fresh or canned, unsweetened)
- 1/2 cup rolled oats
- 1 1/2 cups water
- 1/2 cup low-fat milk or almond milk
- 1 tablespoon honey
- 1 teaspoon ground cinnamon
- 1/4 teaspoon ground nutmeg

Instructions
1. In a medium-sized pot, combine the pumpkin puree, rolled oats, and water.
2. Bring the mixture to a boil, then reduce the heat to a simmer. Cook for 10 minutes, stirring occasionally.
3. Stir in the low-fat milk, honey, ground cinnamon, and ground nutmeg.
4. Continue to cook for another 5 minutes, or until the porridge reaches your desired consistency.
5. Serve warm.

Nutrition Info (per serving)
- Calories: 160
- Protein: 4g
- Carbohydrates: 30g
- Fiber: 4g
- Sugars: 12g
- Fat: 2g
- Saturated Fat: 0.5g
- Sodium: 20mg

Serves
- 2 servings

Cooking Time
- **Total time: 20 minutes**

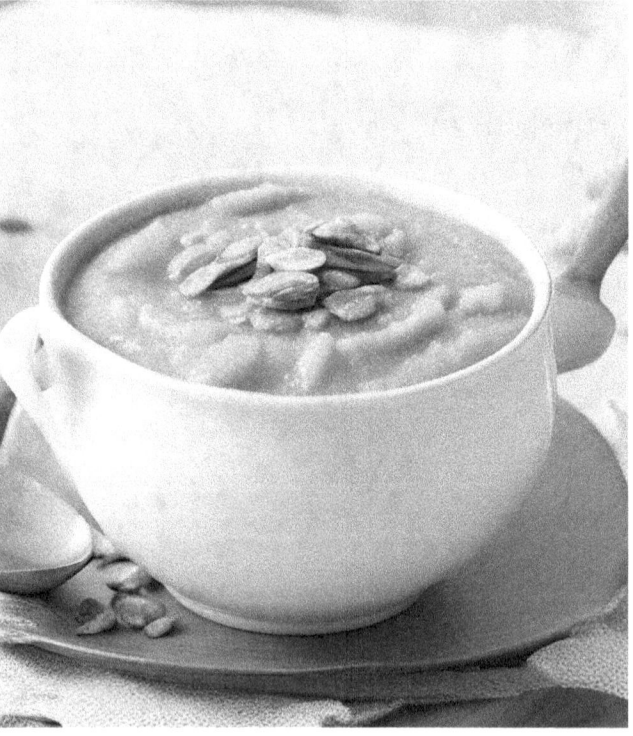

7. Vegetable Omelet

Ingredients
- 2 large eggs
- 1/4 cup low-fat milk
- 1/2 cup spinach, chopped
- 1/4 cup zucchini, grated
- 1/4 cup mushrooms, sliced
- 1 tablespoon olive oil
- 1 tablespoon fresh parsley, chopped

Instructions
1. In a bowl, whisk together the eggs and low-fat milk.
2. Heat the olive oil in a non-stick skillet over medium heat.
3. Add the chopped spinach, grated zucchini, and sliced mushrooms. Cook for 3-4 minutes, until the vegetables are tender.
4. Pour the egg mixture over the vegetables in the skillet.
5. Cook the omelet for 3-4 minutes, until the edges start to set. Gently lift the edges with a spatula and tilt the skillet to allow the uncooked eggs to flow to the edges.
6. Once the omelet is mostly set, sprinkle the chopped parsley over the top.
7. Fold the omelet in half and cook for another 1-2 minutes.
8. Serve warm.

Nutrition Info (per serving)
- Calories: 220
- Protein: 14g
- Carbohydrates: 6g
- Fiber: 2g
- Sugars: 4g
- Fat: 16g
- Saturated Fat: 4g
- Sodium: 140mg

Serves
- **1 serving**

Cooking Time
- **Total time: 15 minutes**

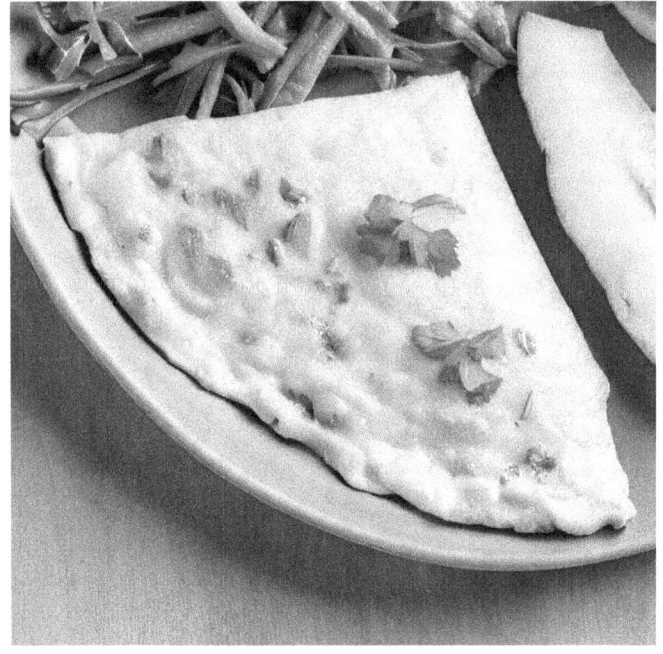

8. Smoothie Bowl

Ingredients
- 1 cup low-fat yogurt
- 1 banana
- 1/2 cup strawberries
- 1/4 cup blueberries
- 1 tablespoon honey
- 1 tablespoon chia seeds
- 1/4 cup granola (optional, make sure it's low in sugar and without added spices)

Instructions
1. In a blender, combine the low-fat yogurt, banana, and strawberries. Blend until smooth.
2. Pour the smoothie into a bowl.
3. Top with blueberries, honey, chia seeds, and granola (if using).
4. Serve immediately.

Nutrition Info (per serving)
- Calories: 250
- Protein: 8g
- Carbohydrates: 45g
- Fiber: 6g
- Sugars: 25g
- Fat: 5g
- Saturated Fat: 2g
- Sodium: 70mg

Serves
- 1 serving

Cooking Time
- **Total time: 10 minutes**

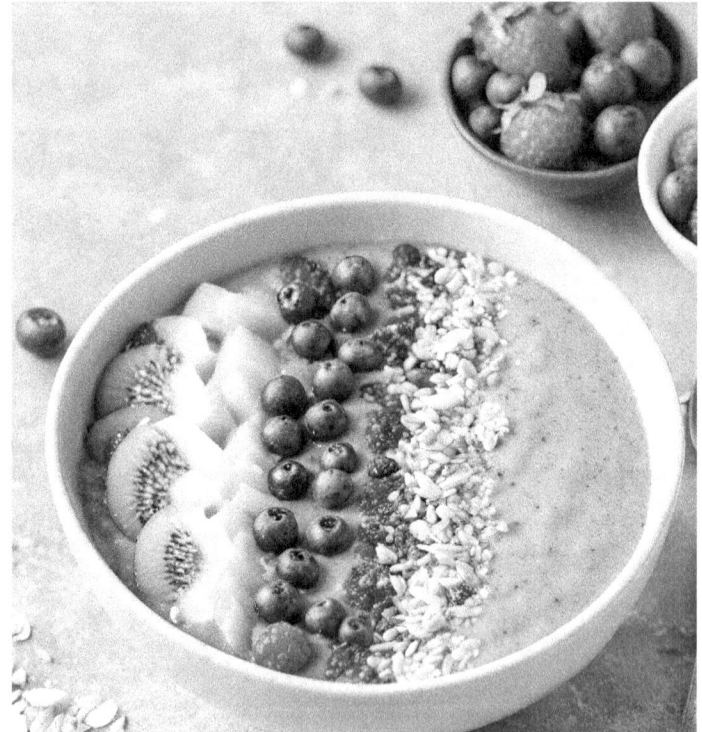

9. Polenta

Ingredients
- 1 cup polenta (cornmeal)
- 4 cups water
- 1 tablespoon olive oil
- 1/4 cup grated Parmesan cheese
- 1 teaspoon dried thyme

Instructions
1. In a medium-sized pot, bring the water to a boil.
2. Gradually whisk in the polenta.
3. Reduce the heat to low and cook, stirring frequently, for about 20-25 minutes, until the polenta is thick and creamy.
4. Remove from heat and stir in the olive oil, grated Parmesan cheese, and dried thyme.
5. Serve warm.

Nutrition Info (per serving)
- Calories: 200
- Protein: 6g
- Carbohydrates: 32g
- Fiber: 3g
- Sugars: 1g
- Fat: 6g
- Saturated Fat: 1.5g
- Sodium: 150mg

Serves
- 4 servings

Cooking Time
- **Total time: 30 minutes**

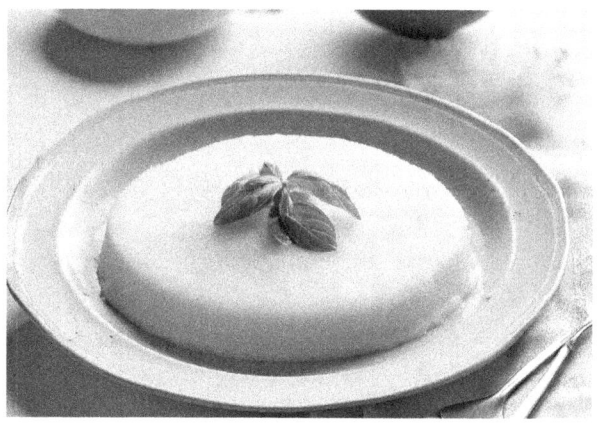

10. Carrot and Ginger Juice

Ingredients

- 4 large carrots, peeled and chopped
- 1-inch piece of fresh ginger, peeled
- 1 apple, cored and chopped (optional for sweetness)
- 1 cup water

Instructions

1. In a blender, combine the carrots, ginger, apple (if using), and water.
2. Blend until smooth.
3. Strain the juice through a fine-mesh sieve or cheesecloth into a jug to remove the pulp.
4. Serve immediately.

Nutrition Info (per serving)

- Calories: 90
- Protein: 1g
- Carbohydrates: 22g
- Fiber: 5g
- Sugars: 13g
- Fat: 0g
- Saturated Fat: 0g
- Sodium: 50mg

Serves

- 2 servings

Cooking Time

- **Total time: 15 minutes**

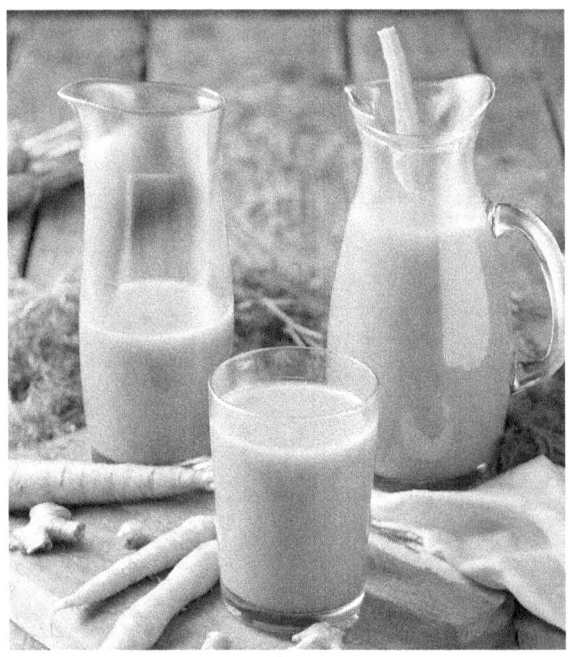

11. Squash Soup

Ingredients
- 1 medium butternut squash, peeled and cubed
- 1 apple, peeled, cored, and chopped
- 4 cups low-sodium vegetable broth
- 1/2 cup low-fat coconut milk
- 1 tablespoon olive oil
- 1 teaspoon ground cinnamon
- 1/4 teaspoon ground nutmeg

Instructions
1. In a large pot, heat the olive oil over medium heat.
2. Add the cubed butternut squash and chopped apple. Cook for 5 minutes, stirring occasionally.
3. Add the vegetable broth, bring to a boil, then reduce the heat and simmer for 20 minutes, or until the squash and apple are tender.
4. Remove from heat and use an immersion blender to puree the soup until smooth. Alternatively, you can transfer the mixture to a blender and blend in batches.
5. Stir in the coconut milk, ground cinnamon, and ground nutmeg.
6. Serve warm.

Nutrition Info (per serving)
- Calories: 180
- Protein: 2g
- Carbohydrates: 30g
- Fiber: 5g
- Sugars: 12g
- Fat: 7g
- Saturated Fat: 4.5g
- Sodium: 150mg

Serves
- 4 servings

Cooking Time
- **Total time: 30 minutes**

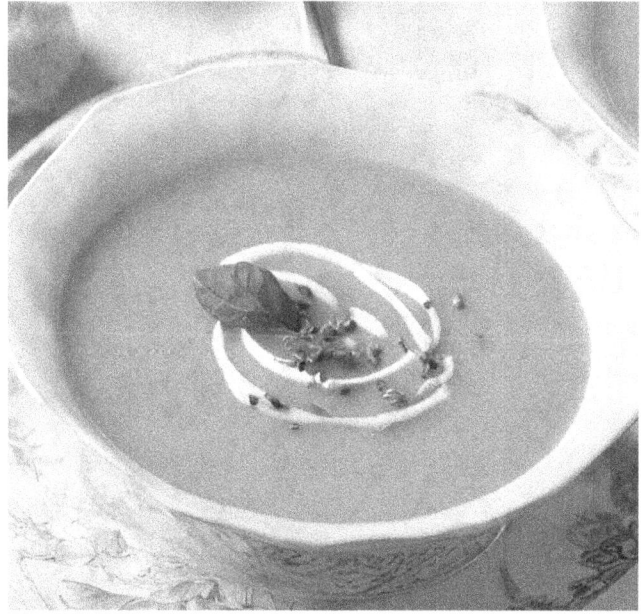

12. Steamed Vegetables

Ingredients
- 1 cup carrots, sliced
- 1 cup green beans, trimmed and cut into 2-inch pieces
- 1 cup zucchini, sliced
- 1 tablespoon olive oil
- 1 teaspoon dried basil

Instructions
1. Fill a large pot with 1-2 inches of water and bring to a boil.
2. Place the carrots, green beans, and zucchini in a steamer basket and set it over the boiling water.
3. Cover and steam the vegetables for about 8-10 minutes, or until they are tender but still crisp.
4. Remove the vegetables from the steamer and place them in a bowl.
5. Drizzle with olive oil and sprinkle with dried basil. Toss to coat.
6. Serve immediately.

Nutrition Info (per serving)
- Calories: 90
- Protein: 2g
- Carbohydrates: 10g
- Fiber: 3g
- Sugars: 5g
- Fat: 5g
- Saturated Fat: 1g
- Sodium: 30mg

Serves
- 2 servings

Cooking Time
- **Total time: 15 minutes**

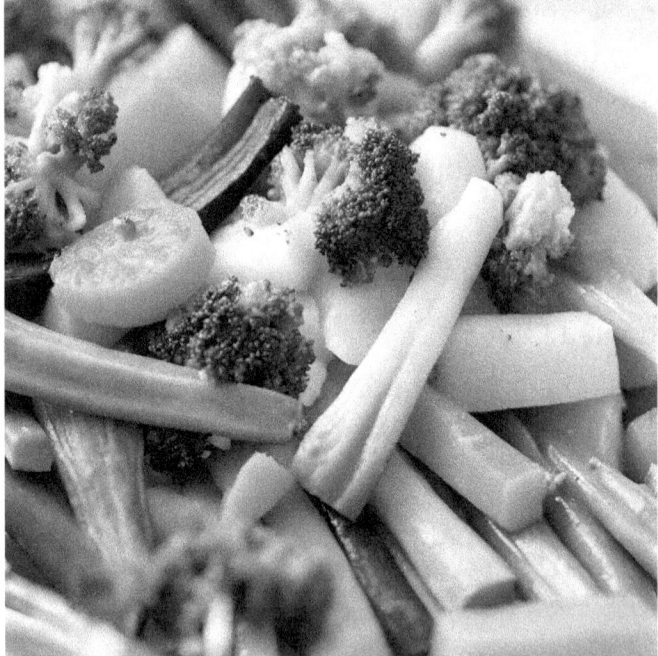

13. Quinoa Salad

Ingredients
- 1 cup quinoa, rinsed
- 2 cups water
- 1/2 cup cucumber, diced
- 1/2 cup cherry tomatoes, halved (if tolerated)
- 1/4 cup feta cheese, crumbled
- 1/4 cup fresh parsley, chopped
- 2 tablespoons olive oil
- 1 tablespoon lemon juice (if tolerated)

Instructions
1. In a medium pot, bring the water to a boil.
2. Add the rinsed quinoa, reduce the heat to low, cover, and simmer for 15 minutes or until the water is absorbed and the quinoa is tender.
3. Remove from heat and let it sit for 5 minutes, then fluff with a fork.
4. In a large bowl, combine the cooked quinoa, cucumber, cherry tomatoes, feta cheese, and parsley.
5. Drizzle with olive oil and lemon juice (if tolerated).
6. Toss gently to combine and serve.

Nutrition Info (per serving)
- Calories: 200
- Protein: 6g
- Carbohydrates: 26g
- Fiber: 4g
- Sugars: 3g
- Fat: 8g
- Saturated Fat: 2g
- Sodium: 140mg

Serves
- 4 servings

Cooking Time
- **Total time: 25 minutes**

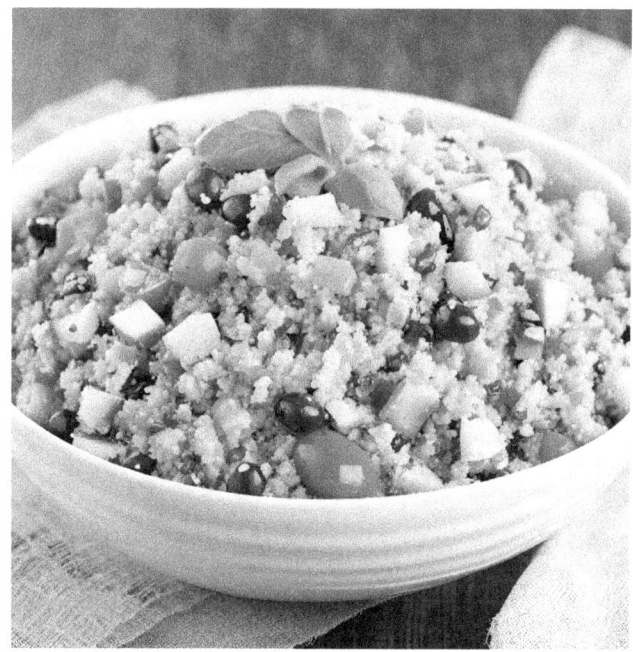

14. Sweet Potato Hash

Ingredients
- 2 medium sweet potatoes, peeled and diced
- 1 small zucchini, diced
- 1/2 cup mushrooms, sliced
- 2 tablespoons olive oil
- 1 teaspoon dried thyme
- 1/2 teaspoon ground paprika

Instructions
1. Heat the olive oil in a large skillet over medium heat.
2. Add the diced sweet potatoes and cook for 10 minutes, stirring occasionally, until they begin to soften.
3. Add the zucchini and mushrooms to the skillet.
4. Sprinkle with dried thyme and ground paprika.
5. Cook for another 10-15 minutes, stirring occasionally, until all the vegetables are tender and lightly browned.
6. Serve warm.

Nutrition Info (per serving)
- Calories: 180
- Protein: 3g
- Carbohydrates: 28g
- Fiber: 5g
- Sugars: 8g
- Fat: 6g
- Saturated Fat: 1g
- Sodium: 50mg

Serves
- 2 servings

Cooking Time
- **Total time: 30 minutes**

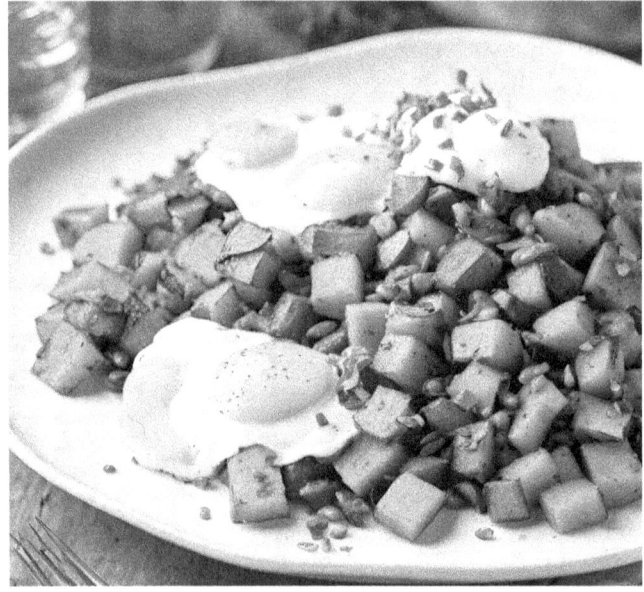

15. Cauliflower Toast

Ingredients
- 1 small head of cauliflower, grated
- 2 large eggs
- 1/2 cup shredded mozzarella cheese
- 1 teaspoon dried oregano
- 1 teaspoon garlic powder
- 1 tablespoon olive oil

Instructions
1. Preheat your oven to 375°F (190°C). Line a baking sheet with parchment paper.
2. Place the grated cauliflower in a microwave-safe bowl and microwave on high for 5 minutes, or until soft. Allow it to cool slightly.
3. Transfer the cauliflower to a clean kitchen towel or cheesecloth. Squeeze out as much moisture as possible.
4. In a large bowl, combine the cauliflower, eggs, shredded mozzarella, dried oregano, and garlic powder. Mix well to form a dough-like consistency.
5. Place the mixture on the prepared baking sheet and shape it into toast-sized rectangles, about 1/2 inch thick.
6. Brush the tops with olive oil.
7. Bake in the preheated oven for 20-25 minutes, or until golden brown and firm.
8. Remove from the oven and let cool slightly before serving.

Nutrition Info (per serving)
- Calories: 110
- Protein: 8g
- Carbohydrates: 4g
- Fiber: 2g
- Sugars: 2g
- Fat: 7g
- Saturated Fat: 3g
- Sodium: 150mg

Serves
- **4 servings**

Cooking Time
- **Total time: 35 minutes**

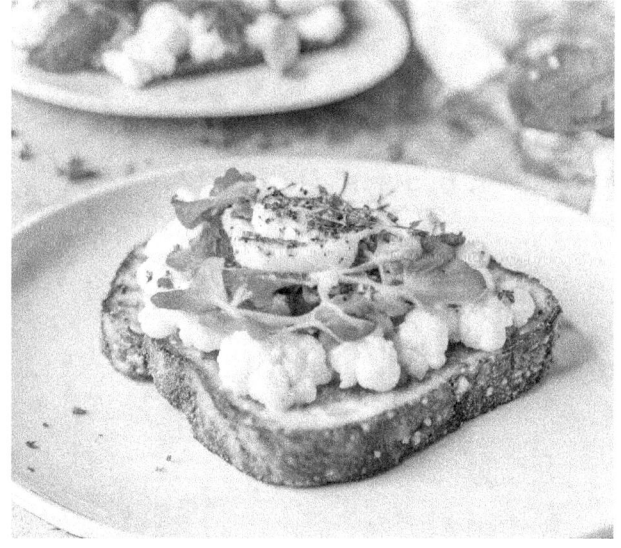

16. Almond Rice Porridge

Ingredients
- 1 cup white rice
- 4 cups almond milk
- 1/4 cup sliced almonds
- 2 tablespoons honey
- 1 teaspoon ground cinnamon
- 1 teaspoon vanilla extract

Instructions
1. Rinse the rice under cold water until the water runs clear.
2. In a medium pot, bring the almond milk to a gentle boil.
3. Add the rice, reduce the heat to low, and cover. Simmer for about 20-25 minutes, stirring occasionally, until the rice is tender and the mixture is creamy.
4. Stir in the sliced almonds, honey, ground cinnamon, and vanilla extract.
5. Cook for an additional 5 minutes, stirring frequently.
6. Serve warm.

Nutrition Info (per serving)
- Calories: 250
- Protein: 6g
- Carbohydrates: 45g
- Fiber: 2g
- Sugars: 14g
- Fat: 5g
- Saturated Fat: 1g
- Sodium: 60mg

Serves
- **4 servings**

Cooking Time
- **Total time: 35 minutes**

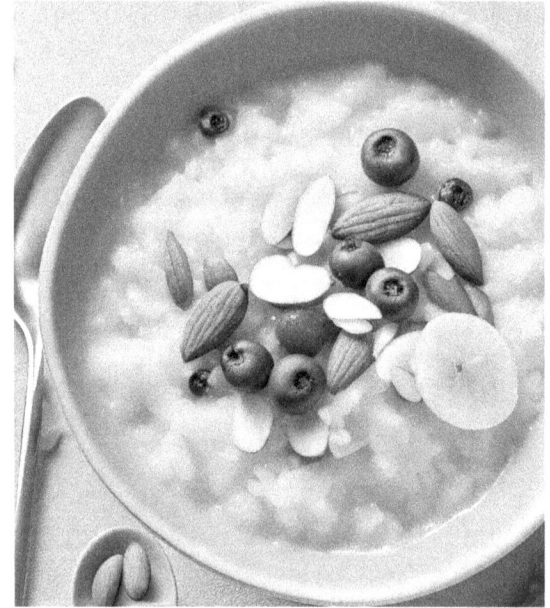

17. Soft Boiled Eggs

Ingredients
- 4 large eggs
- Water for boiling

Instructions
1. Bring a medium pot of water to a gentle boil.
2. Carefully lower the eggs into the boiling water using a spoon.
3. Boil the eggs for 6 minutes for soft-boiled eggs with a slightly runny yolk.
4. Remove the eggs from the boiling water and place them in a bowl of ice water to stop the cooking process.
5. Let the eggs cool for about 2 minutes, then gently peel them.
6. Serve warm.

Nutrition Info (per serving)
- Calories: 70
- Protein: 6g
- Carbohydrates: 1g
- Fiber: 0g
- Sugars: 1g
- Fat: 5g
- Saturated Fat: 1.5g
- Sodium: 65mg

Serves
- 4 servings

Cooking Time
- **Total time: 10 minutes**

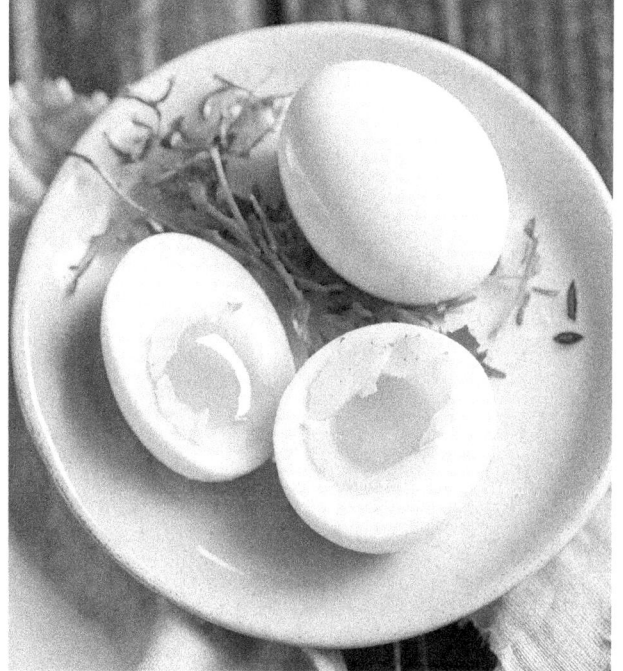

18. Barley Soup

Ingredients
- 1 cup pearl barley
- 6 cups low-sodium vegetable broth
- 2 carrots, diced
- 2 celery stalks, diced
- 1 small zucchini, diced
- 1 tablespoon olive oil
- 1 teaspoon dried thyme
- 1 teaspoon dried basil

Instructions
1. Rinse the barley under cold water.
2. In a large pot, heat the olive oil over medium heat.
3. Add the diced carrots, celery, and zucchini. Cook for about 5 minutes, stirring occasionally.
4. Add the rinsed barley and cook for an additional 2 minutes, stirring to coat the barley with the oil and vegetables.
5. Pour in the vegetable broth and bring to a boil.
6. Reduce the heat to low, add the dried thyme and dried basil, and simmer for about 45 minutes, or until the barley is tender.
7. Serve warm.

Nutrition Info (per serving)
- Calories: 200
- Protein: 4g
- Carbohydrates: 40g
- Fiber: 6g
- Sugars: 6g
- Fat: 3g
- Saturated Fat: 0.5g
- Sodium: 250mg

Serves
- 4 servings

Cooking Time
- **Total time: 1 hour**

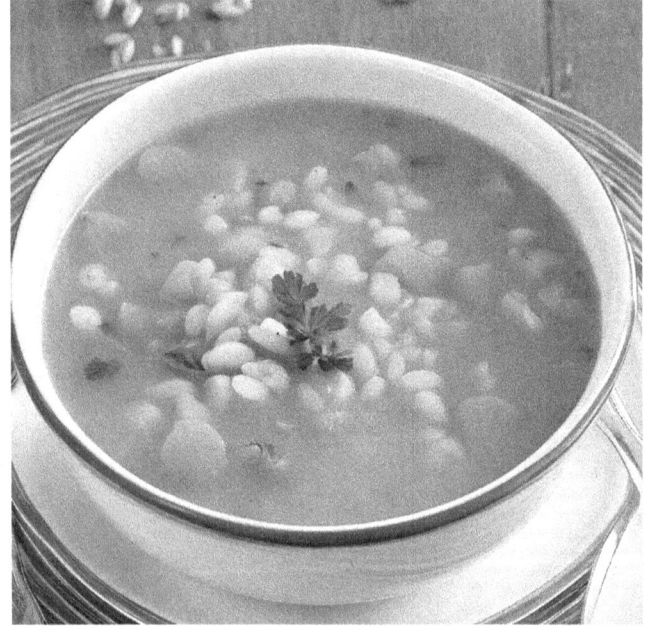

19. Omelet with Herbs

Ingredients
- 2 large eggs
- 1/4 cup low-fat milk
- 1 tablespoon olive oil
- 1 tablespoon fresh parsley, chopped
- 1 tablespoon fresh chives, chopped
- 1 tablespoon fresh dill, chopped

Instructions
1. In a bowl, whisk together the eggs and low-fat milk until well combined.
2. Heat the olive oil in a non-stick skillet over medium heat.
3. Pour the egg mixture into the skillet and cook until the edges start to set, about 2-3 minutes.
4. Sprinkle the chopped parsley, chives, and dill evenly over the eggs.
5. Continue to cook for another 2-3 minutes until the omelet is fully set.
6. Fold the omelet in half and slide it onto a plate.
7. Serve warm.

Nutrition Info (per serving)
- Calories: 220
- Protein: 12g
- Carbohydrates: 2g
- Fiber: 1g
- Sugars: 1g
- Fat: 18g
- Saturated Fat: 4g
- Sodium: 120mg

Serves
- 1 serving

Cooking Time
- **Total time: 10 minutes**

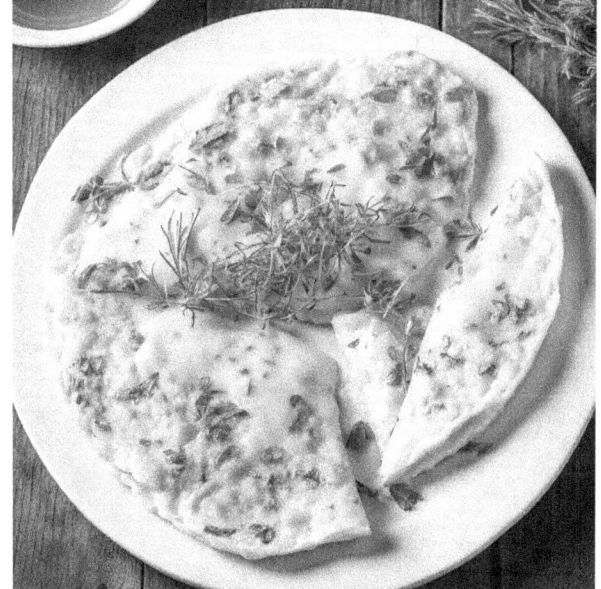

20. Zucchini Bread

Ingredients
- 1 1/2 cups grated zucchini
- 1 cup whole wheat flour
- 1 cup all-purpose flour
- 1/2 cup honey
- 1/2 cup applesauce
- 2 large eggs
- 1/2 cup vegetable oil
- 1 teaspoon baking powder
- 1 teaspoon baking soda
- 1 teaspoon ground cinnamon
- 1/4 teaspoon ground nutmeg
- 1/2 cup chopped walnuts (optional)

Instructions
1. Preheat your oven to 350°F (175°C). Grease and flour a 9x5-inch loaf pan.
2. In a large bowl, mix together the whole wheat flour, all-purpose flour, baking powder, baking soda, ground cinnamon, and ground nutmeg.
3. In another bowl, beat the eggs and mix in the honey, applesauce, vegetable oil, and grated zucchini.
4. Combine the wet ingredients with the dry ingredients and stir until just combined. Fold in the chopped walnuts if using.
5. Pour the batter into the prepared loaf pan.
6. Bake for 50-60 minutes, or until a toothpick inserted into the center comes out clean.
7. Let the bread cool in the pan for 10 minutes, then transfer to a wire rack to cool completely.
8. Slice and serve.

Nutrition Info (per serving)
- Calories: 180
- Protein: 4g
- Carbohydrates: 26g
- Fiber: 2g
- Sugars: 12g
- Fat: 7g
- Saturated Fat: 1g
- Sodium: 120mg

Serves
- 12 servings

Cooking Time
- **Total time: 70 minutes**

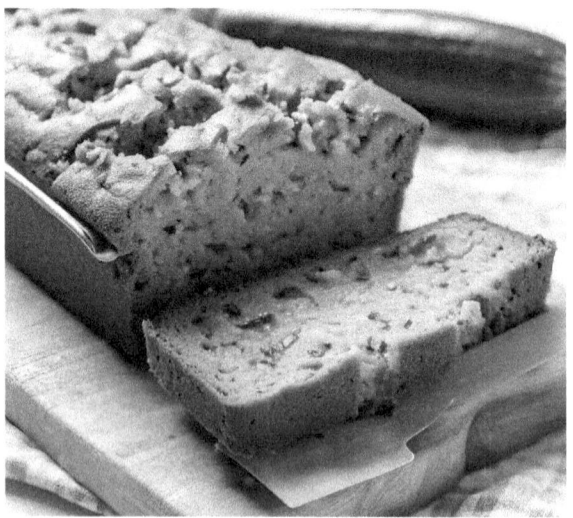

21. Millet Porridge

Ingredients
- 1 cup millet
- 3 cups water
- 1 cup low-fat milk or almond milk
- 1 tablespoon honey
- 1 teaspoon ground cinnamon
- 1/4 teaspoon ground nutmeg

Instructions
1. Rinse the millet under cold water.
2. In a medium-sized pot, bring the water to a boil.
3. Add the millet, reduce the heat to low, cover, and simmer for about 20 minutes, or until the millet is tender and the water is absorbed.
4. Stir in the milk, honey, ground cinnamon, and ground nutmeg.
5. Cook for an additional 5 minutes, stirring frequently, until the porridge reaches your desired consistency.
6. Serve warm.

Nutrition Info (per serving)
- Calories: 210
- Protein: 5g
- Carbohydrates: 38g
- Fiber: 4g
- Sugars: 8g
- Fat: 3g
- Saturated Fat: 1g
- Sodium: 20mg

Serves
- **4 servings**

Cooking Time
- **Total time: 30 minutes**

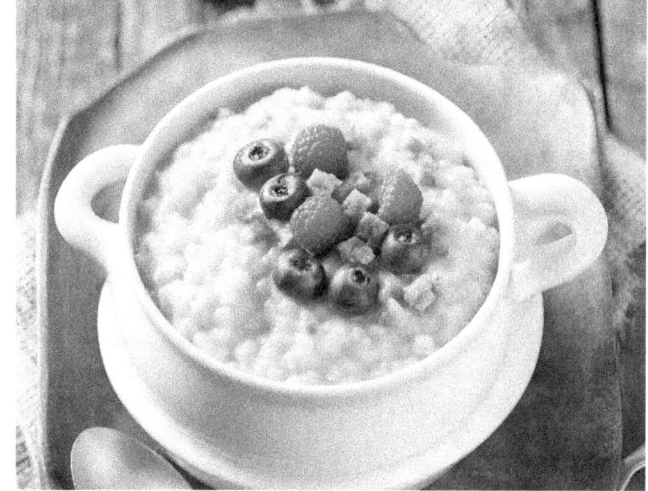

22. Pear Smoothie

Ingredients
- 1 ripe pear, cored and chopped
- 1/2 banana
- 1 cup low-fat yogurt
- 1/2 cup almond milk
- 1 tablespoon honey
- 1/2 teaspoon ground flaxseed

Instructions
1. In a blender, combine the pear, banana, low-fat yogurt, almond milk, honey, and ground flaxseed.
2. Blend on high until smooth and creamy.
3. Pour the smoothie into a glass and serve immediately.

Nutrition Info (per serving)
- Calories: 180
- Protein: 6g
- Carbohydrates: 34g
- Fiber: 4g
- Sugars: 22g
- Fat: 3g
- Saturated Fat: 1g
- Sodium: 70mg

Serves
- 1 serving

Cooking Time
- **Total time: 5 minutes**

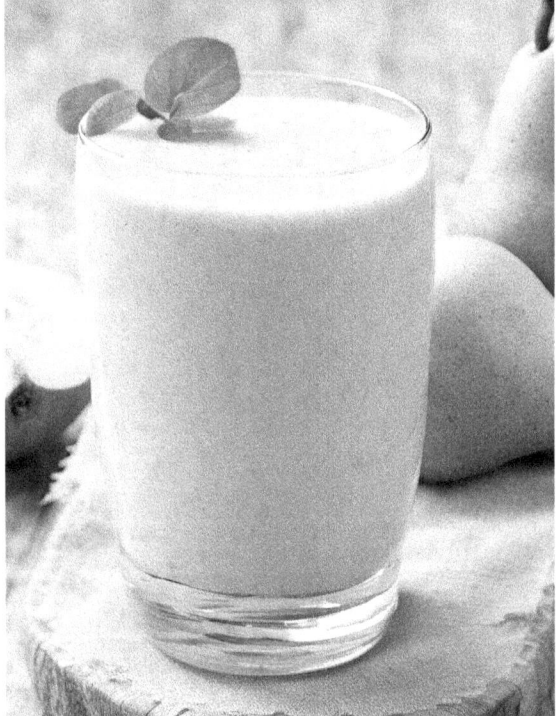

23. Buckwheat Pancakes

Ingredients
- 1 cup buckwheat flour
- 1 cup low-fat milk or almond milk
- 1 large egg
- 2 tablespoons honey
- 1 teaspoon baking powder
- 1/2 teaspoon ground cinnamon
- 1/4 teaspoon ground nutmeg
- 1 tablespoon olive oil

Instructions
1. In a large bowl, whisk together the buckwheat flour, baking powder, ground cinnamon, and ground nutmeg.
2. In another bowl, whisk together the milk, egg, and honey until well combined.
3. Pour the wet ingredients into the dry ingredients and mix until just combined.
4. Heat a non-stick skillet over medium heat and add a little olive oil.
5. Pour 1/4 cup of batter onto the skillet for each pancake. Cook until bubbles form on the surface, then flip and cook until the other side is golden brown, about 2-3 minutes per side.
6. Repeat with the remaining batter.
7. Serve warm with additional honey or fruit, if desired.

Nutrition Info (per serving)
- Calories: 180
- Protein: 5g
- Carbohydrates: 30g
- Fiber: 4g
- Sugars: 8g
- Fat: 5g
- Saturated Fat: 1g
- Sodium: 120mg

Serves
- **4 servings**

Cooking Time
- **Total time: 20 minutes**

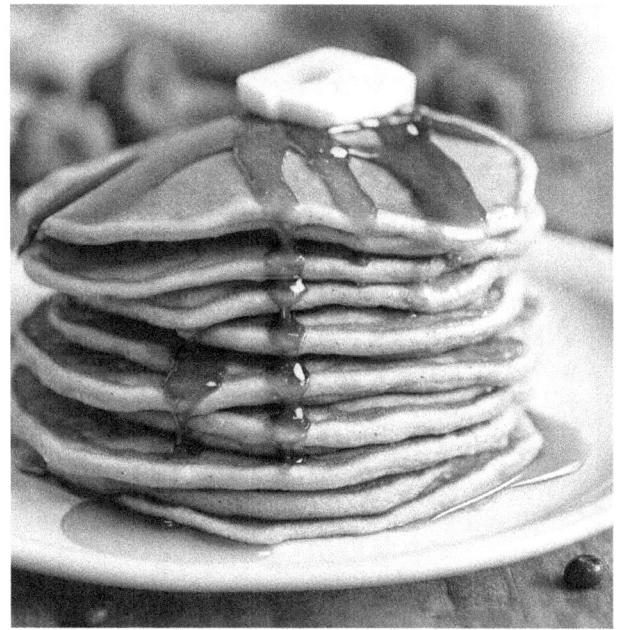

24. Rye Bread Sandwich

Ingredients
- 4 slices of rye bread
- 4 ounces low-fat turkey or chicken breast, thinly sliced
- 4 slices of cucumber
- 4 slices of low-fat cheese
- 1 tablespoon mayonnaise (optional)
- 1 tablespoon Dijon mustard (optional)
- Fresh lettuce leaves

Instructions
1. Toast the rye bread slices lightly if desired.
2. Spread a thin layer of mayonnaise and Dijon mustard on each slice of bread (if using).
3. Layer the turkey or chicken breast, cucumber slices, cheese, and lettuce on two slices of bread.
4. Top with the remaining slices of bread to form sandwiches.
5. Cut the sandwiches in half and serve immediately.

Nutrition Info (per serving)
- Calories: 250
- Protein: 16g
- Carbohydrates: 32g
- Fiber: 4g
- Sugars: 4g
- Fat: 7g
- Saturated Fat: 2g
- Sodium: 500mg

Serves
- 2 servings

Cooking Time
- **Total time: 10 minutes**

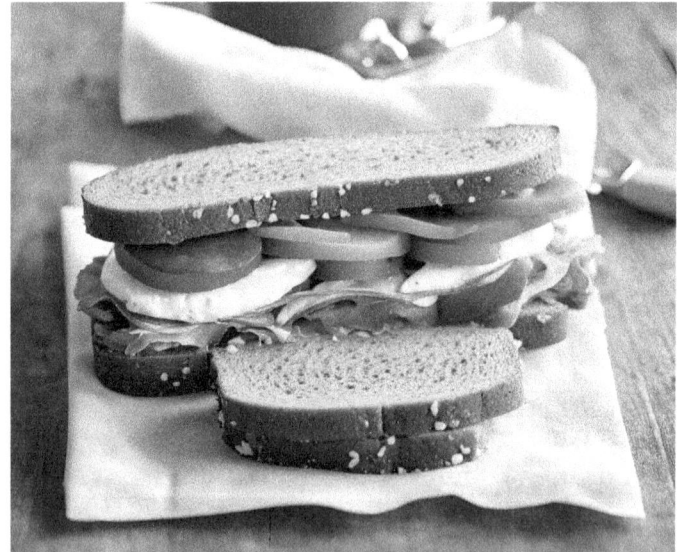

25. Basil and Spinach Smoothie

Ingredients
- 1 cup fresh spinach leaves
- 1/4 cup fresh basil leaves
- 1 ripe banana
- 1 cup almond milk
- 1 tablespoon honey
- 1 tablespoon chia seeds
- 1/2 teaspoon vanilla extract

Instructions
1. In a blender, combine the spinach, basil, banana, almond milk, honey, chia seeds, and vanilla extract.
2. Blend on high until smooth and creamy.
3. Pour the smoothie into a glass and serve immediately.

Nutrition Info (per serving)
- Calories: 180
- Protein: 4g
- Carbohydrates: 35g
- Fiber: 5g
- Sugars: 22g
- Fat: 4g
- Saturated Fat: 0.5g
- Sodium: 80mg

Serves
- 1 serving

Cooking Time
- **Total time: 5 minutes**

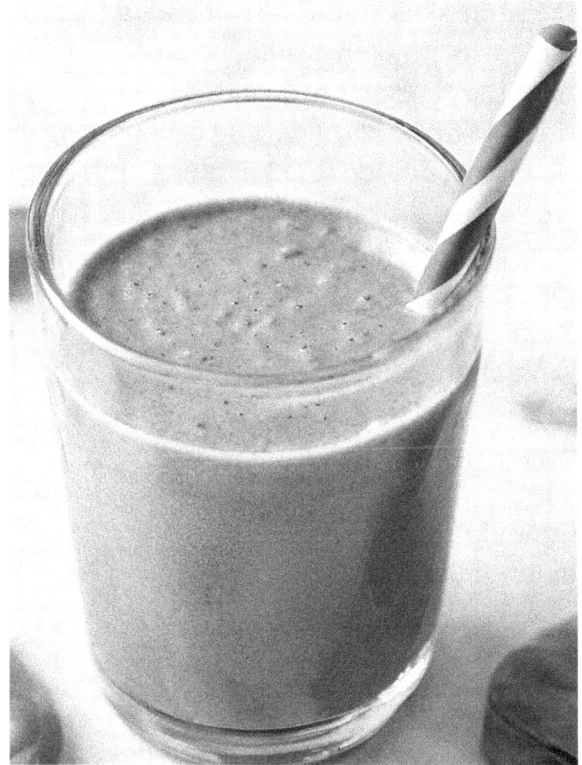

Poultry Recipes

1. Chicken and Carrot Noodles
Ingredients
- 2 boneless, skinless chicken breasts
- 4 large carrots, peeled and spiralized into noodles
- 2 tablespoons olive oil
- 1 cup low-sodium chicken broth
- 1 tablespoon fresh parsley, chopped
- 1 teaspoon dried thyme
- 1/2 teaspoon ground ginger

Instructions
1. Heat 1 tablespoon of olive oil in a large skillet over medium heat.
2. Add the chicken breasts and cook for about 6-7 minutes on each side, or until fully cooked. Remove from the skillet and let rest for 5 minutes before slicing.
3. In the same skillet, add the remaining tablespoon of olive oil.
4. Add the carrot noodles and cook for 3-4 minutes, until they are tender.
5. Pour in the chicken broth and add the sliced chicken back into the skillet.
6. Sprinkle with dried thyme and ground ginger, stirring to combine.
7. Cook for an additional 2-3 minutes, until everything is heated through.
8. Serve warm, garnished with fresh parsley.

Nutrition Info (per serving)
- Calories: 300
- Protein: 30g
- Carbohydrates: 15g
- Fiber: 5g
- Sugars: 8g
- Fat: 12g
- Saturated Fat: 2g
- Sodium: 350mg

Serves
- 2 servings

Cooking Time
- **Total time: 20 minutes**

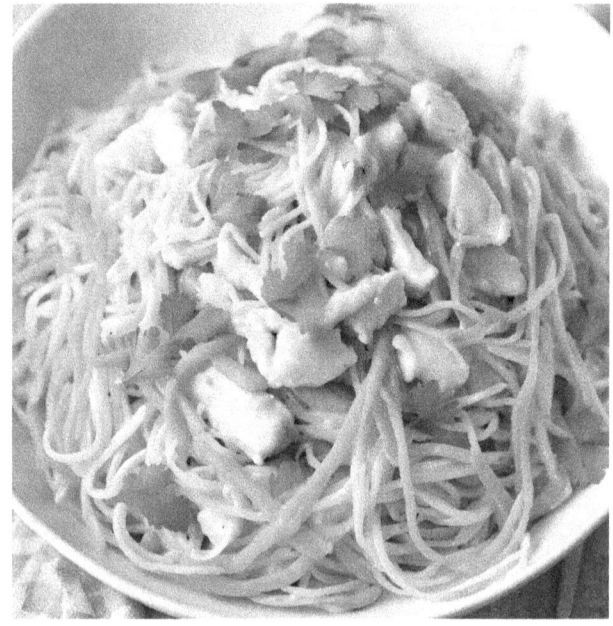

2. Turkey and Oat Porridge

Ingredients
- 1 cup ground turkey
- 1 cup rolled oats
- 2 cups low-sodium chicken broth
- 1/2 cup carrots, finely diced
- 1/2 cup zucchini, finely diced
- 1 tablespoon olive oil
- 1 teaspoon dried basil

Instructions
1. Heat the olive oil in a large pot over medium heat.
2. Add the ground turkey and cook until fully browned, breaking it up with a spoon as it cooks.
3. Add the carrots and zucchini, and cook for an additional 5 minutes until the vegetables are tender.
4. Stir in the rolled oats and pour in the chicken broth.
5. Bring the mixture to a boil, then reduce the heat and simmer for 10-15 minutes, stirring occasionally, until the oats are cooked and the porridge is thickened.
6. Stir in the dried basil.
7. Serve warm.

Nutrition Info (per serving)
- Calories: 280
- Protein: 25g
- Carbohydrates: 30g
- Fiber: 5g
- Sugars: 2g
- Fat: 9g
- Saturated Fat: 2g
- Sodium: 320mg

Serves
- 2 servings

Cooking Time
- **Total time: 25 minutes**

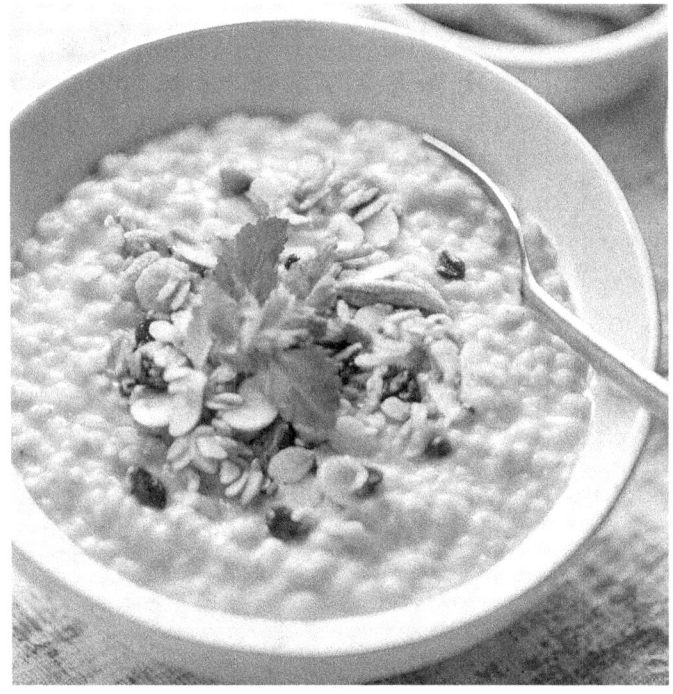

3. Chicken Cauliflower Fried Rice

Ingredients
- 2 boneless, skinless chicken breasts, diced
- 1 medium head of cauliflower, grated into rice-sized pieces
- 1/2 cup peas
- 1/2 cup carrots, diced
- 2 large eggs, lightly beaten
- 2 tablespoons olive oil
- 2 tablespoons low-sodium soy sauce
- 1 teaspoon ground ginger
- 1 tablespoon fresh chives, chopped

Instructions
1. Heat 1 tablespoon of olive oil in a large skillet or wok over medium heat.
2. Add the diced chicken and cook until fully cooked, about 6-7 minutes. Remove from the skillet and set aside.
3. In the same skillet, add the remaining tablespoon of olive oil.
4. Add the grated cauliflower, peas, and carrots, and cook for 5-7 minutes, stirring frequently, until the vegetables are tender.
5. Push the vegetables to one side of the skillet and pour the beaten eggs onto the other side. Scramble the eggs until fully cooked, then mix them with the vegetables.
6. Add the cooked chicken back into the skillet.
7. Pour in the low-sodium soy sauce and sprinkle with ground ginger. Stir everything together until well combined and heated through.
8. Serve warm, garnished with fresh chives.

Nutrition Info (per serving)
- Calories: 320
- Protein: 30g
- Carbohydrates: 15g
- Fiber: 5g
- Sugars: 4g
- Fat: 15g
- Saturated Fat: 3g
- Sodium: 400mg

Serves
- 2 servings

Cooking Time
- **Total time: 25 minutes**

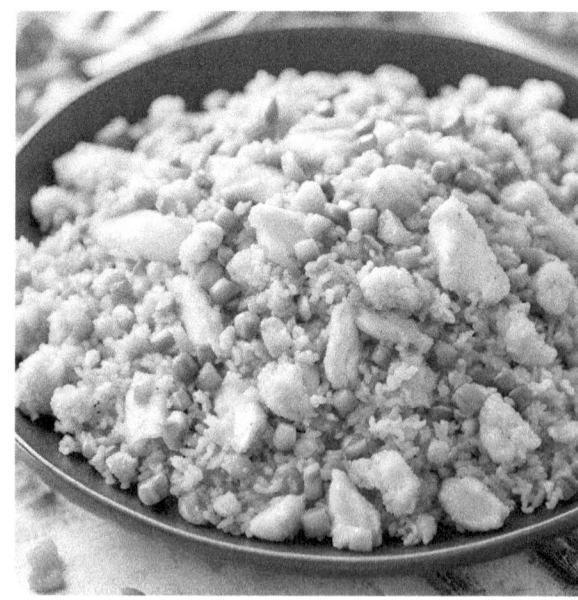

4. Baked Turkey and Eggplant

Ingredients
- 2 boneless, skinless turkey breasts
- 1 large eggplant, sliced into 1/2-inch rounds
- 2 tablespoons olive oil
- 1 teaspoon dried thyme
- 1 teaspoon dried basil
- 1/2 cup low-fat mozzarella cheese, shredded

Instructions
1. Preheat your oven to 375°F (190°C).
2. Place the eggplant slices on a baking sheet and brush both sides with olive oil.
3. Sprinkle the dried thyme and dried basil evenly over the eggplant slices.
4. Lay the turkey breasts on top of the eggplant slices.
5. Sprinkle the shredded mozzarella cheese over the turkey breasts.
6. Bake in the preheated oven for 25-30 minutes, or until the turkey is fully cooked and the cheese is melted and golden.
7. Serve warm.

Nutrition Info (per serving)
- Calories: 300
- Protein: 35g
- Carbohydrates: 10g
- Fiber: 4g
- Sugars: 5g
- Fat: 14g
- Saturated Fat: 4g
- Sodium: 160mg

Serves
- 2 servings

Cooking Time
- **Total time: 35 minutes**

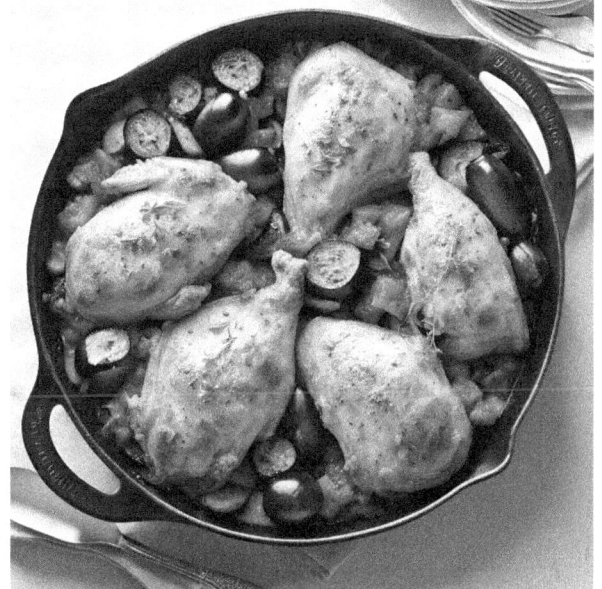

5. Chicken and Avocado Salad

Ingredients
- 2 boneless, skinless chicken breasts, grilled and sliced
- 2 cups mixed greens (spinach, arugula, lettuce)
- 1 ripe avocado, sliced
- 1/2 cup cherry tomatoes, halved (if tolerated)
- 1/4 cup shredded carrots
- 2 tablespoons olive oil
- 1 tablespoon lemon juice (if tolerated)
- 1 teaspoon dried oregano

Instructions
1. In a large salad bowl, combine the mixed greens, cherry tomatoes, and shredded carrots.
2. Add the grilled and sliced chicken breast and avocado slices on top.
3. In a small bowl, whisk together the olive oil, lemon juice, and dried oregano.
4. Drizzle the dressing over the salad and toss gently to combine.
5. Serve immediately.

Nutrition Info (per serving)
- Calories: 350
- Protein: 30g
- Carbohydrates: 12g
- Fiber: 7g
- Sugars: 3g
- Fat: 22g
- Saturated Fat: 4g
- Sodium: 120mg

Serves
- 2 servings

Cooking Time
- **Total time: 15 minutes (plus grilling time for the chicken)**

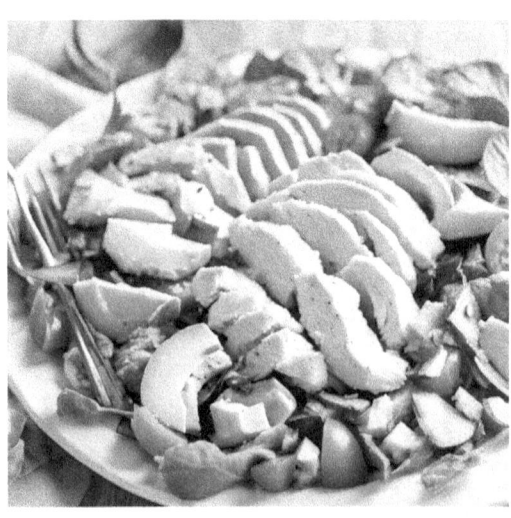

6. Turkey and Potato Soup

Ingredients
- 1 cup ground turkey
- 2 large potatoes, peeled and diced
- 2 carrots, diced
- 2 celery stalks, diced
- 4 cups low-sodium chicken broth
- 1 tablespoon olive oil
- 1 teaspoon dried thyme
- 1 teaspoon dried parsley

Instructions
1. Heat the olive oil in a large pot over medium heat.
2. Add the ground turkey and cook until fully browned, breaking it up with a spoon as it cooks.
3. Add the diced potatoes, carrots, and celery to the pot.
4. Pour in the low-sodium chicken broth and add the dried thyme and dried parsley.
5. Bring the soup to a boil, then reduce the heat and simmer for 20-25 minutes, or until the vegetables are tender.
6. Serve warm.

Nutrition Info (per serving)
- Calories: 250
- Protein: 20g
- Carbohydrates: 30g
- Fiber: 5g
- Sugars: 5g
- Fat: 8g
- Saturated Fat: 2g
- Sodium: 200mg

Serves
- 4 servings

Cooking Time
- **Total time: 35 minutes**

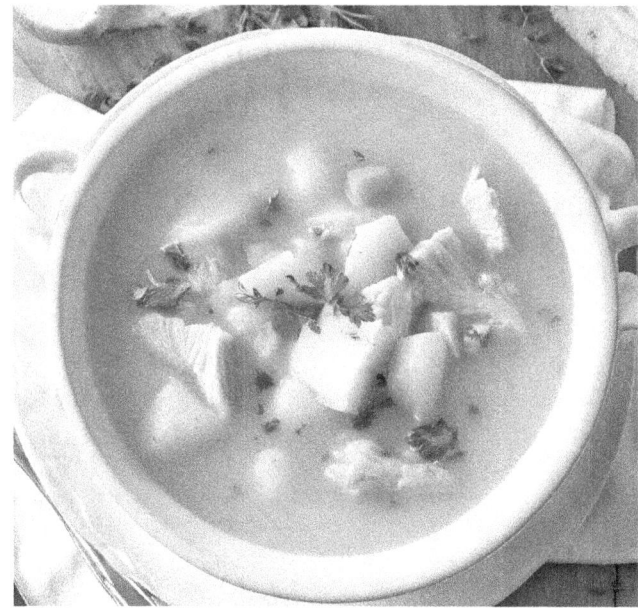

7. Steam-Fried Chicken Drumsticks

Ingredients
- 6 chicken drumsticks, skin removed
- 1 tablespoon olive oil
- 1 teaspoon dried rosemary
- 1 teaspoon ground paprika
- 1/2 cup low-sodium chicken broth

Instructions
1. Heat the olive oil in a large skillet over medium heat.
2. Add the chicken drumsticks and cook for about 5 minutes on each side, until browned.
3. Sprinkle the dried rosemary and ground paprika evenly over the drumsticks.
4. Pour the chicken broth into the skillet and cover with a lid.
5. Reduce the heat to low and let the drumsticks steam for 15-20 minutes, or until fully cooked and tender.
6. Remove the lid and increase the heat to medium-high to evaporate any remaining liquid, allowing the drumsticks to get a crispy exterior.
7. Serve warm.

Nutrition Info (per serving)
- Calories: 220
- Protein: 25g
- Carbohydrates: 2g
- Fiber: 0g
- Sugars: 0g
- Fat: 12g
- Saturated Fat: 3g
- Sodium: 150mg

Serves
- 3 servings

Cooking Time
- **Total time: 30 minutes**

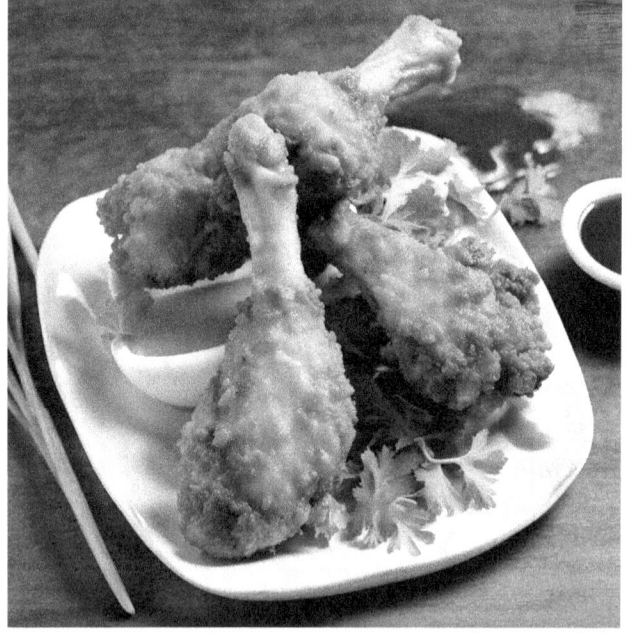

8. Turkey Vegetable Loaf

Ingredients

- 1 pound ground turkey
- 1/2 cup grated zucchini
- 1/2 cup grated carrots
- 1/4 cup finely chopped spinach
- 1/2 cup rolled oats
- 1/4 cup low-fat milk
- 1 large egg
- 1 teaspoon dried thyme
- 1 teaspoon dried basil

Instructions

1. Preheat your oven to 350°F (175°C). Lightly grease a loaf pan.
2. In a large bowl, combine the ground turkey, grated zucchini, grated carrots, chopped spinach, rolled oats, low-fat milk, egg, dried thyme, and dried basil.
3. Mix until well combined.
4. Press the mixture evenly into the prepared loaf pan.
5. Bake in the preheated oven for 50-60 minutes, or until the internal temperature reaches 165°F (74°C) and the top is golden brown.
6. Let the loaf rest for 5 minutes before slicing and serving.

Nutrition Info (per serving)

- Calories: 220
- Protein: 25g
- Carbohydrates: 12g
- Fiber: 2g
- Sugars: 3g
- Fat: 9g
- Saturated Fat: 2g
- Sodium: 85mg

Serves

- **4 servings**

Cooking Time

- **Total time: 1 hour 10 minutes**

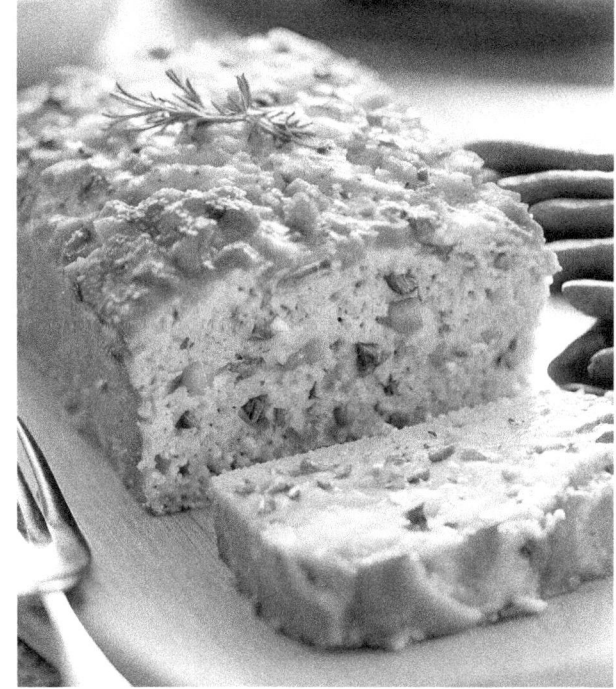

9. Slow Cooked Chicken with Oats

Ingredients
- 2 boneless, skinless chicken breasts
- 1 cup rolled oats
- 4 cups low-sodium chicken broth
- 1 cup diced carrots
- 1 cup diced celery
- 1 teaspoon dried rosemary
- 1 teaspoon dried thyme

Instructions
1. Place the chicken breasts in the slow cooker.
2. Add the rolled oats, chicken broth, diced carrots, diced celery, dried rosemary, and dried thyme.
3. Stir to combine all ingredients.
4. Cover and cook on low for 6-8 hours, or until the chicken is tender and fully cooked.
5. Shred the chicken with two forks and stir it back into the oat mixture.
6. Serve warm.

Nutrition Info (per serving)
- Calories: 240
- Protein: 24g
- Carbohydrates: 26g
- Fiber: 4g
- Sugars: 3g
- Fat: 5g
- Saturated Fat: 1g
- Sodium: 150mg

Serves
- 4 servings

Cooking Time
- **Total time: 6-8 hours**

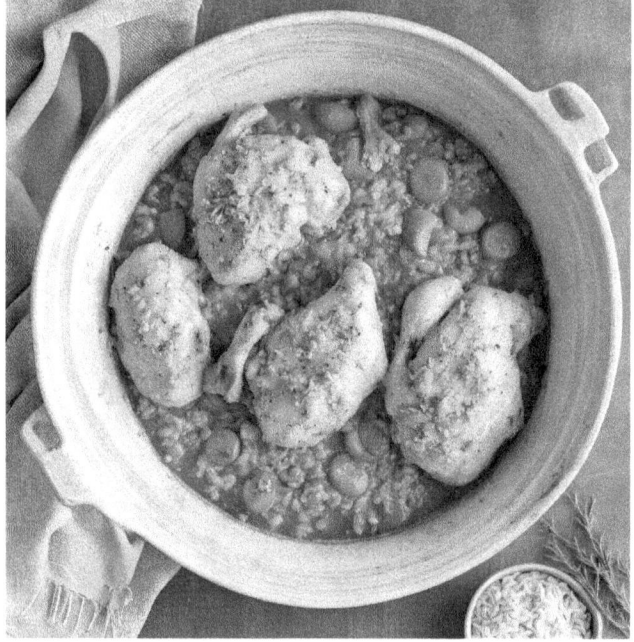

10. Herbed Turkey Steaks

Ingredients
- 4 turkey steaks (about 4 ounces each)
- 2 tablespoons olive oil
- 1 teaspoon dried oregano
- 1 teaspoon dried basil
- 1 teaspoon dried parsley
- 1/2 teaspoon ground paprika

Instructions
1. Preheat your grill or skillet to medium-high heat.
2. In a small bowl, combine the olive oil, dried oregano, dried basil, dried parsley, and ground paprika.
3. Brush the mixture evenly over both sides of the turkey steaks.
4. Grill or cook the turkey steaks in the skillet for about 5-7 minutes on each side, or until the internal temperature reaches 165°F (74°C).
5. Remove from heat and let the steaks rest for 5 minutes before serving.

Nutrition Info (per serving)
- Calories: 210
- Protein: 28g
- Carbohydrates: 1g
- Fiber: 0g
- Sugars: 0g
- Fat: 10g
- Saturated Fat: 2g
- Sodium: 60mg

Serves
- 4 servings

Cooking Time
- **Total time: 20 minutes**

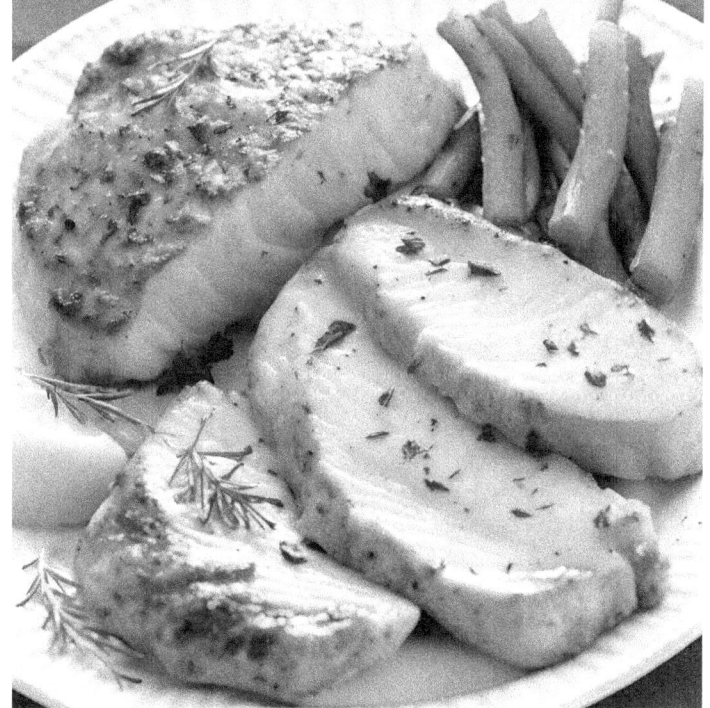

11. Chicken Paillard

Ingredients
- 2 boneless, skinless chicken breasts
- 2 tablespoons olive oil
- 1 teaspoon dried thyme
- 1 teaspoon dried basil
- 1/2 teaspoon ground paprika
- 1 tablespoon lemon juice (if tolerated)
- Fresh parsley, chopped (for garnish)

Instructions
1. Place the chicken breasts between two pieces of plastic wrap and pound them to an even thickness using a meat mallet.
2. In a small bowl, mix together the olive oil, dried thyme, dried basil, ground paprika, and lemon juice.
3. Brush the mixture evenly over both sides of the chicken breasts.
4. Heat a non-stick skillet over medium-high heat.
5. Cook the chicken breasts for 3-4 minutes on each side, or until fully cooked and golden brown.
6. Remove from the skillet and let rest for a few minutes before serving.
7. Garnish with chopped parsley and serve warm.

Nutrition Info (per serving)
- Calories: 250
- Protein: 28g
- Carbohydrates: 1g
- Fiber: 0g
- Sugars: 0g
- Fat: 14g
- Saturated Fat: 2g
- Sodium: 80mg

Serves
- 2 servings

Cooking Time
- **Total time: 15 minutes**

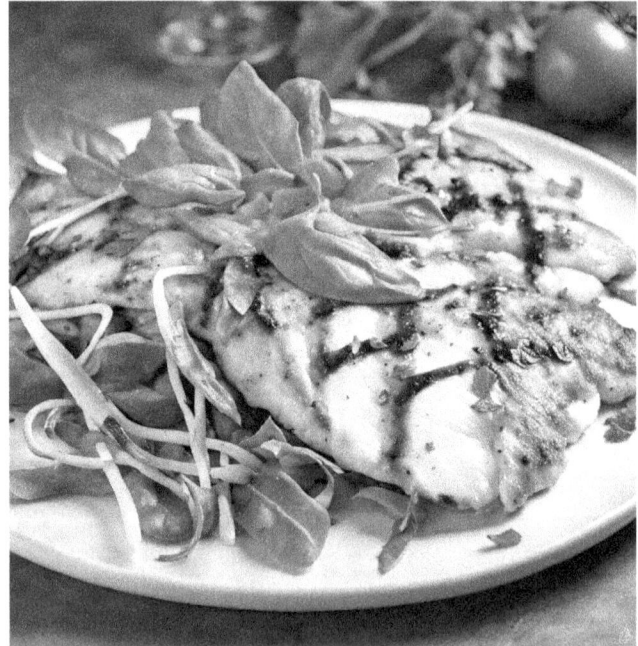

12. Turkey Spinach Meatloaf

Ingredients

- 1 pound ground turkey
- 1 cup fresh spinach, chopped
- 1/2 cup rolled oats
- 1/4 cup low-fat milk
- 1 large egg
- 1 teaspoon dried thyme
- 1 teaspoon dried basil

Instructions

1. Preheat your oven to 350°F (175°C). Lightly grease a loaf pan.
2. In a large bowl, combine the ground turkey, chopped spinach, rolled oats, low-fat milk, egg, dried thyme, and dried basil.
3. Mix until well combined.
4. Press the mixture evenly into the prepared loaf pan.
5. Bake in the preheated oven for 50-60 minutes, or until the internal temperature reaches 165°F (74°C) and the top is golden brown.
6. Let the meatloaf rest for 5 minutes before slicing and serving.

Nutrition Info (per serving)

- Calories: 200
- Protein: 24g
- Carbohydrates: 10g
- Fiber: 2g
- Sugars: 1g
- Fat: 7g
- Saturated Fat: 2g
- Sodium: 75mg

Serves

- **4 servings**

Cooking Time

- **Total time: 1 hour 10 minutes**

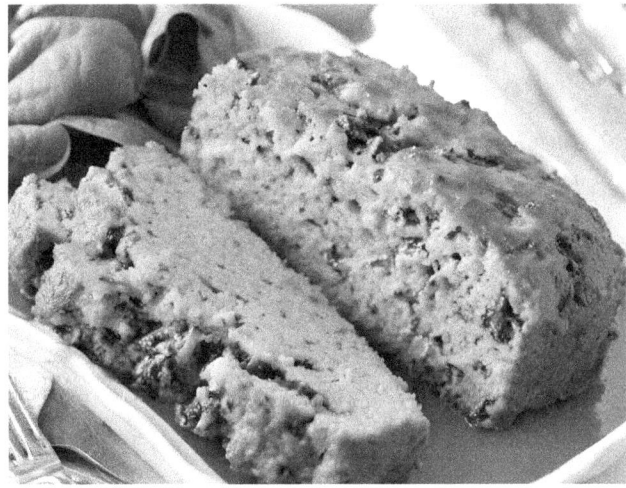

13. Chicken and Parsnip Stew

Ingredients
- 2 boneless, skinless chicken breasts, diced
- 2 parsnips, peeled and diced
- 2 carrots, peeled and diced
- 1 cup green beans, cut into 1-inch pieces
- 4 cups low-sodium chicken broth
- 1 tablespoon olive oil
- 1 teaspoon dried thyme
- 1 teaspoon dried rosemary

Instructions
1. Heat the olive oil in a large pot over medium heat.
2. Add the diced chicken breasts and cook until browned, about 5-7 minutes.
3. Add the parsnips, carrots, and green beans to the pot.
4. Pour in the low-sodium chicken broth and add the dried thyme and dried rosemary.
5. Bring the stew to a boil, then reduce the heat and simmer for 20-25 minutes, or until the vegetables are tender.
6. Serve warm.

Nutrition Info (per serving)
- Calories: 240
- Protein: 22g
- Carbohydrates: 20g
- Fiber: 5g
- Sugars: 6g
- Fat: 9g
- Saturated Fat: 2g
- Sodium: 180mg

Serves
- **4 servings**

Cooking Time
- **Total time: 35 minutes**

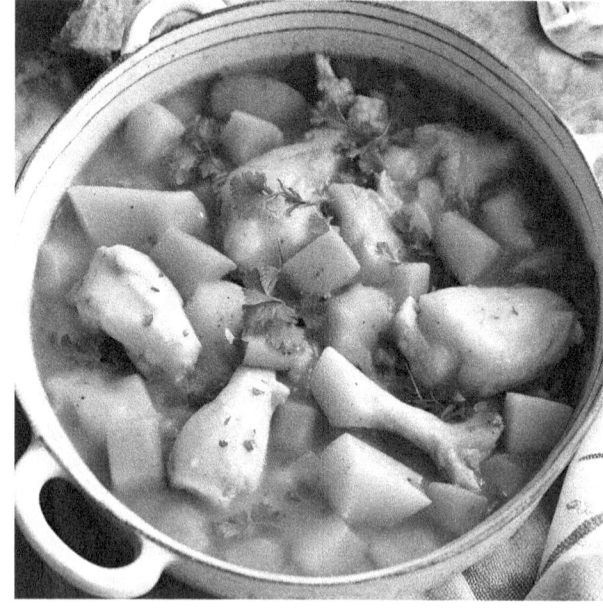

14. Stuffed Chicken Breast

Ingredients
- 2 boneless, skinless chicken breasts
- 1/2 cup fresh spinach, chopped
- 1/4 cup low-fat mozzarella cheese, shredded
- 1 tablespoon olive oil
- 1 teaspoon dried basil

Instructions
1. Preheat your oven to 375°F (190°C).
2. Using a sharp knife, carefully cut a pocket into each chicken breast.
3. In a small bowl, mix together the chopped spinach and shredded mozzarella cheese.
4. Stuff each chicken breast with the spinach and cheese mixture.
5. Secure the openings with toothpicks if needed.
6. Brush the chicken breasts with olive oil and sprinkle with dried basil.
7. Place the chicken breasts in a baking dish and bake in the preheated oven for 25-30 minutes, or until fully cooked and the cheese is melted and bubbly.
8. Remove from the oven and let rest for a few minutes before serving.

Nutrition Info (per serving)
- Calories: 280
- Protein: 32g
- Carbohydrates: 2g
- Fiber: 1g
- Sugars: 0g
- Fat: 16g
- Saturated Fat: 4g
- Sodium: 120mg

Serves
- 2 servings

Cooking Time
- **Total time: 35 minutes**

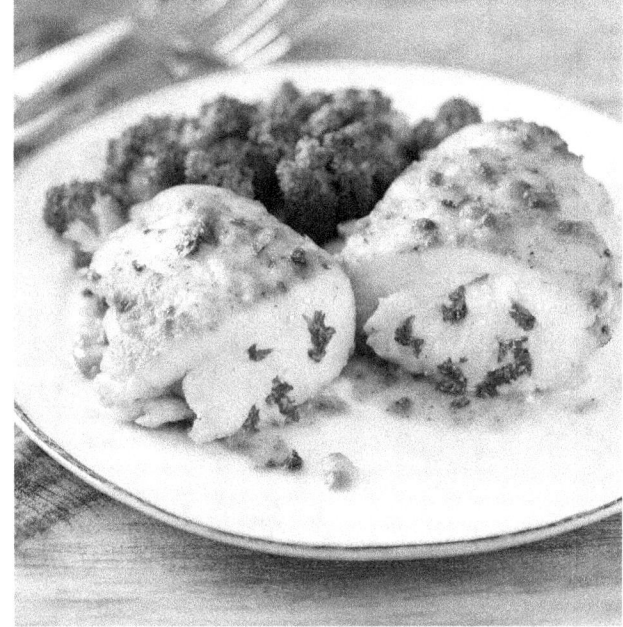

15. Turkey and Carrot Patties

Ingredients
- 1 pound ground turkey
- 1 cup grated carrots
- 1/4 cup rolled oats
- 1 large egg
- 1 teaspoon dried thyme
- 1 teaspoon dried basil
- 2 tablespoons olive oil

Instructions
1. In a large bowl, combine the ground turkey, grated carrots, rolled oats, egg, dried thyme, and dried basil. Mix until well combined.
2. Form the mixture into patties, about 2 inches in diameter.
3. Heat the olive oil in a large skillet over medium heat.
4. Cook the patties for about 5-6 minutes on each side, or until fully cooked and golden brown.
5. Remove from the skillet and drain on paper towels.
6. Serve warm.

Nutrition Info (per serving)
- Calories: 230
- Protein: 25g
- Carbohydrates: 10g
- Fiber: 2g
- Sugars: 2g
- Fat: 10g
- Saturated Fat: 2g
- Sodium: 80mg

Serves
- 4 servings

Cooking Time
- **Total time: 20 minutes**

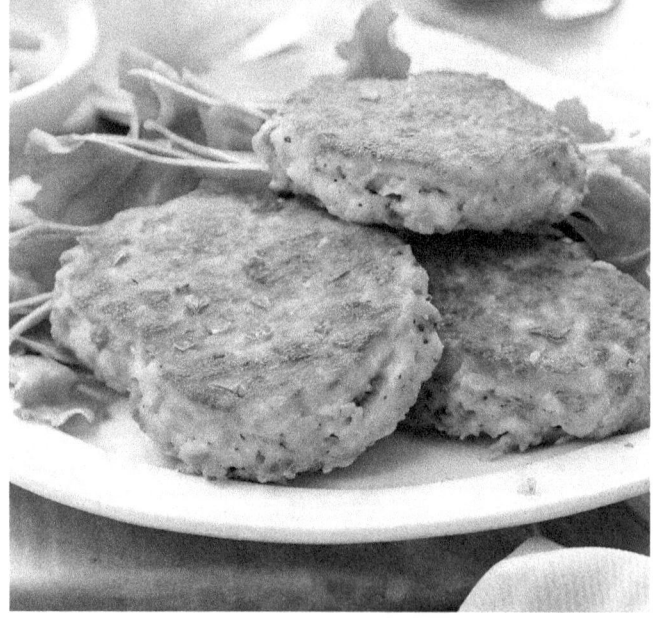

16. Chicken and Peas Pilaf

Ingredients
- 2 boneless, skinless chicken breasts, diced
- 1 cup basmati rice
- 2 cups low-sodium chicken broth
- 1 cup frozen peas, thawed
- 1 tablespoon olive oil
- 1 teaspoon dried basil
- 1 teaspoon dried thyme

Instructions
1. Heat the olive oil in a large pot over medium heat.
2. Add the diced chicken and cook until browned, about 5-7 minutes.
3. Add the basmati rice and cook for an additional 2 minutes, stirring frequently.
4. Pour in the chicken broth and add the dried basil and dried thyme.
5. Bring to a boil, then reduce the heat, cover, and simmer for 15 minutes.
6. Stir in the thawed peas, cover, and cook for another 5 minutes, or until the rice is tender and the liquid is absorbed.
7. Serve warm.

Nutrition Info (per serving)
- Calories: 300
- Protein: 28g
- Carbohydrates: 35g
- Fiber: 4g
- Sugars: 2g
- Fat: 6g
- Saturated Fat: 1g
- Sodium: 160mg

Serves
- 4 servings

Cooking Time
- **Total time: 30 minutes**

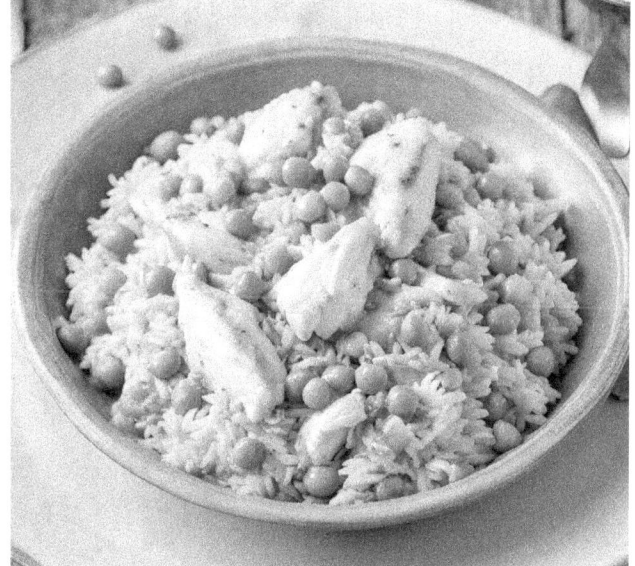

17. Chicken and Potato Bake

Ingredients
- 2 boneless, skinless chicken breasts, diced
- 4 medium potatoes, peeled and diced
- 1 cup carrots, diced
- 1/2 cup low-fat mozzarella cheese, shredded
- 1 tablespoon olive oil
- 1 teaspoon dried rosemary
- 1 teaspoon dried thyme

Instructions
1. Preheat your oven to 375°F (190°C). Lightly grease a baking dish.
2. In a large bowl, combine the diced chicken, diced potatoes, and diced carrots.
3. Drizzle with olive oil and sprinkle with dried rosemary and dried thyme. Toss to coat.
4. Spread the mixture evenly in the prepared baking dish.
5. Cover with foil and bake for 25 minutes.
6. Remove the foil, sprinkle with shredded mozzarella cheese, and bake for an additional 10-15 minutes, or until the chicken is fully cooked and the cheese is melted and golden brown.
7. Serve warm.

Nutrition Info (per serving)
- Calories: 350
- Protein: 30g
- Carbohydrates: 35g
- Fiber: 5g
- Sugars: 3g
- Fat: 12g
- Saturated Fat: 4g
- Sodium: 180mg

Serves
- 4 servings

Cooking Time
- **Total time: 40 minutes**

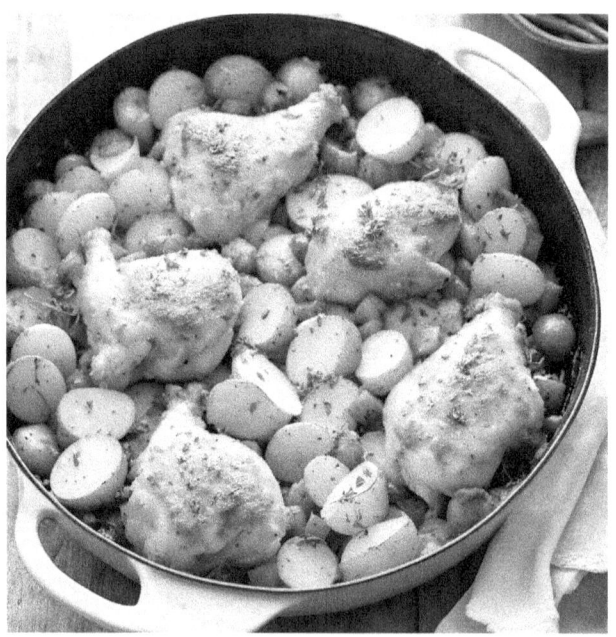

18. Turkey Quinoa Salad

Ingredients
- 1 cup cooked quinoa
- 1 cup cooked turkey breast, diced
- 1/2 cup cucumber, diced
- 1/2 cup cherry tomatoes, halved (if tolerated)
- 1/4 cup feta cheese, crumbled
- 2 tablespoons olive oil
- 1 tablespoon lemon juice (if tolerated)
- 1 teaspoon dried oregano

Instructions
1. In a large bowl, combine the cooked quinoa, diced turkey breast, diced cucumber, cherry tomatoes, and feta cheese.
2. In a small bowl, whisk together the olive oil, lemon juice, and dried oregano.
3. Pour the dressing over the salad and toss gently to combine.
4. Serve immediately or refrigerate until ready to eat.

Nutrition Info (per serving)
- Calories: 300
- Protein: 25g
- Carbohydrates: 20g
- Fiber: 3g
- Sugars: 3g
- Fat: 15g
- Saturated Fat: 4g
- Sodium: 200mg

Serves
- 4 servings

Cooking Time
- **Total time: 20 minutes**

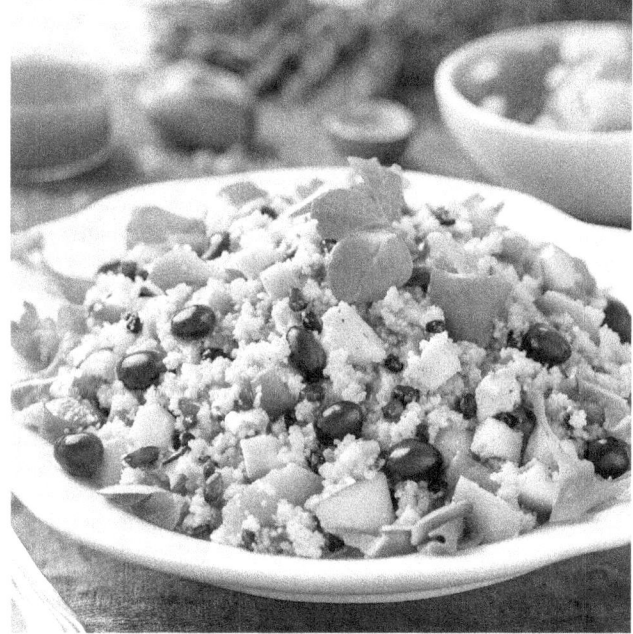

19. Baked Chicken and Mushrooms

Ingredients
- 2 boneless, skinless chicken breasts
- 1 cup mushrooms, sliced
- 1/2 cup low-fat mozzarella cheese, shredded
- 2 tablespoons olive oil
- 1 teaspoon dried thyme
- 1 teaspoon dried rosemary

Instructions
1. Preheat your oven to 375°F (190°C). Lightly grease a baking dish.
2. Place the chicken breasts in the baking dish.
3. In a bowl, toss the sliced mushrooms with olive oil, dried thyme, and dried rosemary.
4. Spread the mushroom mixture over the chicken breasts.
5. Sprinkle the shredded mozzarella cheese over the top.
6. Cover with foil and bake for 25 minutes.
7. Remove the foil and bake for an additional 10-15 minutes, or until the chicken is fully cooked and the cheese is melted and golden brown.
8. Serve warm.

Nutrition Info (per serving)
- Calories: 280
- Protein: 30g
- Carbohydrates: 3g
- Fiber: 1g
- Sugars: 1g
- Fat: 16g
- Saturated Fat: 5g
- Sodium: 180mg

Serves
- **2 servings**

Cooking Time
- **Total time: 40 minutes**

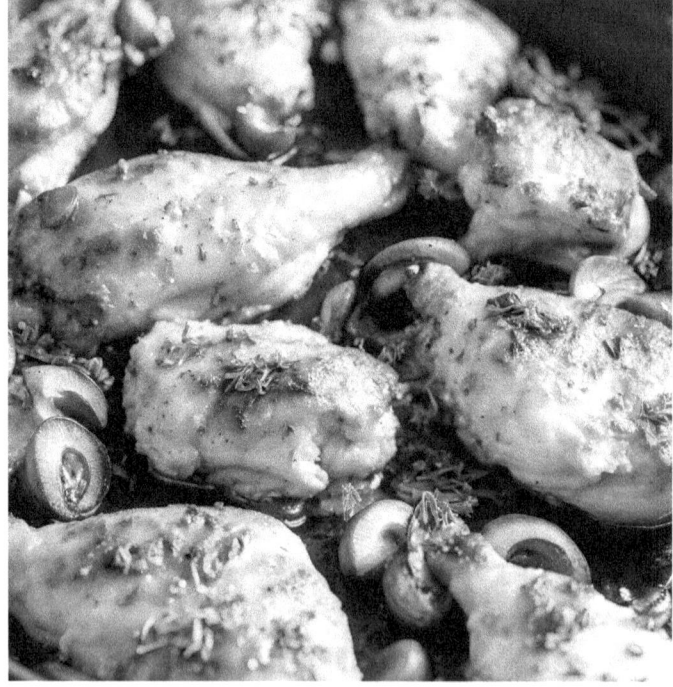

20. Turkey and Squash Skillet

Ingredients
- 1 pound ground turkey
- 2 cups butternut squash, peeled and diced
- 1 cup green beans, cut into 1-inch pieces
- 2 tablespoons olive oil
- 1 teaspoon dried basil
- 1 teaspoon dried thyme

Instructions
1. Heat the olive oil in a large skillet over medium heat.
2. Add the ground turkey and cook until browned, about 5-7 minutes.
3. Add the diced butternut squash and green beans to the skillet.
4. Sprinkle with dried basil and dried thyme.
5. Cover and cook for 10-15 minutes, stirring occasionally, until the vegetables are tender and the turkey is fully cooked.
6. Serve warm.

Nutrition Info (per serving)
- Calories: 250
- Protein: 24g
- Carbohydrates: 18g
- Fiber: 4g
- Sugars: 4g
- Fat: 10g
- Saturated Fat: 2g
- Sodium: 120mg

Serves
- 4 servings

Cooking Time
- **Total time: 25 minutes**

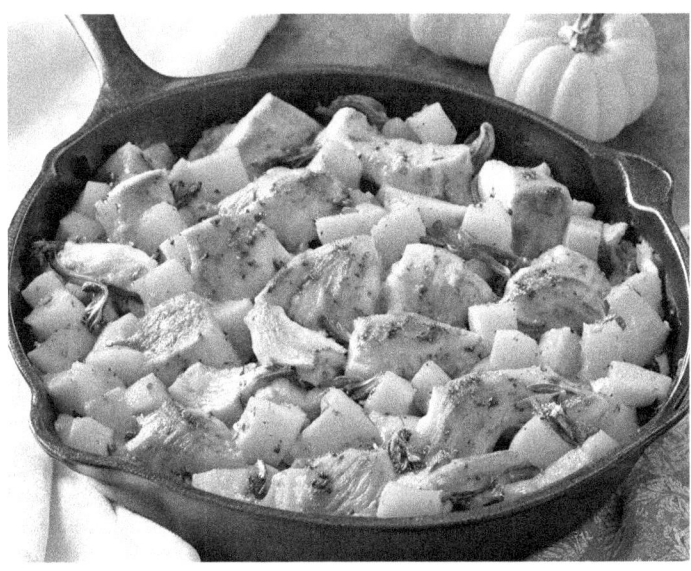

21. Chicken Porridge

Ingredients
- 1 cup cooked chicken breast, shredded
- 1 cup rice
- 4 cups low-sodium chicken broth
- 1 cup carrots, diced
- 1 tablespoon olive oil
- 1 teaspoon dried thyme
- 1 teaspoon ground ginger

Instructions
1. Heat the olive oil in a large pot over medium heat.
2. Add the rice and cook for 2 minutes, stirring frequently.
3. Pour in the chicken broth and add the diced carrots, dried thyme, and ground ginger.
4. Bring to a boil, then reduce the heat and simmer for 20-25 minutes, or until the rice is tender and the mixture is thickened.
5. Stir in the shredded chicken and cook for an additional 5 minutes.
6. Serve warm.

Nutrition Info (per serving)
- Calories: 220
- Protein: 20g
- Carbohydrates: 28g
- Fiber: 2g
- Sugars: 2g
- Fat: 5g
- Saturated Fat: 1g
- Sodium: 150mg

Serves
- 4 servings

Cooking Time
- **Total time: 35 minutes**

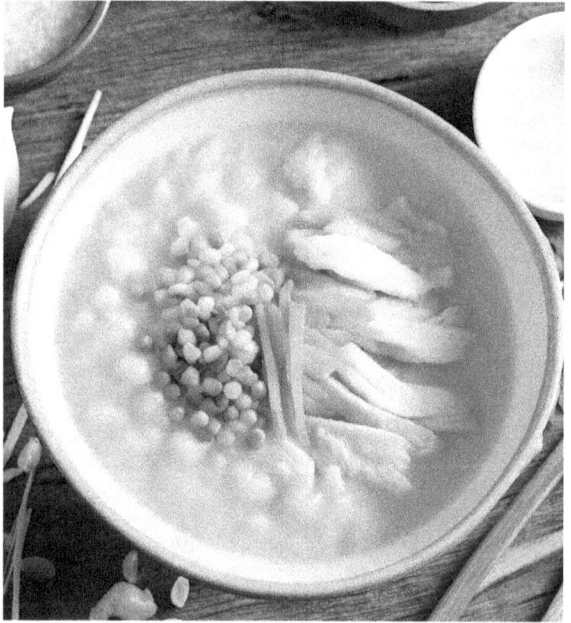

22. Chicken and Zucchini Boats

Ingredients
- 2 boneless, skinless chicken breasts, diced
- 4 large zucchinis, halved lengthwise and seeds scooped out
- 1 cup low-fat mozzarella cheese, shredded
- 2 tablespoons olive oil
- 1 teaspoon dried oregano
- 1 teaspoon dried basil

Instructions
1. Preheat your oven to 375°F (190°C). Lightly grease a baking dish.
2. Heat 1 tablespoon of olive oil in a skillet over medium heat.
3. Add the diced chicken and cook until browned, about 5-7 minutes.
4. Remove the chicken from the heat and set aside.
5. Brush the zucchini halves with the remaining tablespoon of olive oil and sprinkle with dried oregano and dried basil.
6. Fill each zucchini half with the cooked chicken and place them in the baking dish.
7. Sprinkle the shredded mozzarella cheese over the top.
8. Cover with foil and bake for 20 minutes.
9. Remove the foil and bake for an additional 10-15 minutes, or until the zucchinis are tender and the cheese is melted and golden brown.
10. Serve warm.

Nutrition Info (per serving)
- Calories: 270
- Protein: 30g
- Carbohydrates: 6g
- Fiber: 2g
- Sugars: 4g
- Fat: 14g
- Saturated Fat: 4g
- Sodium: 160mg

Serves
- **4 servings**

Cooking Time
- **Total time: 35 minutes**

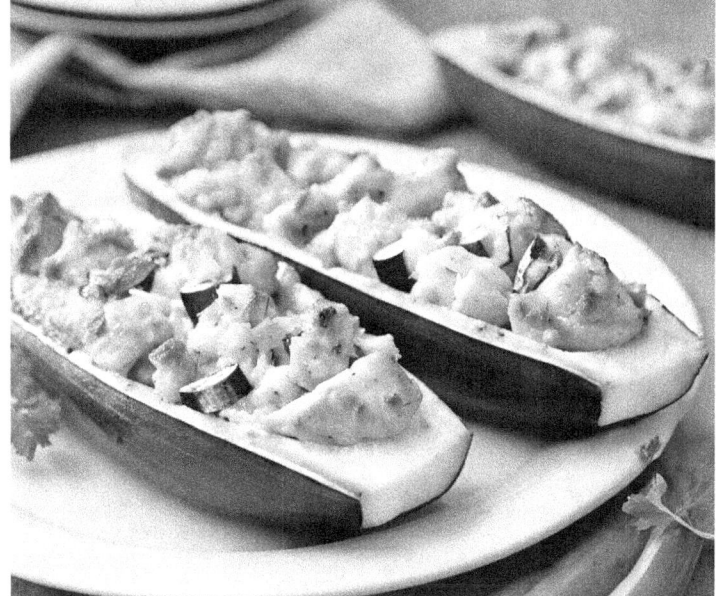

23. Turkey and Sweet Potato Hash

Ingredients
- 1 pound ground turkey
- 2 medium sweet potatoes, peeled and diced
- 1 cup green beans, trimmed and cut into 1-inch pieces
- 1 tablespoon olive oil
- 1 teaspoon dried thyme
- 1 teaspoon dried basil

Instructions
1. Heat the olive oil in a large skillet over medium heat.
2. Add the ground turkey and cook until browned, about 5-7 minutes.
3. Add the diced sweet potatoes and cook for an additional 10 minutes, stirring occasionally, until the sweet potatoes begin to soften.
4. Add the green beans, dried thyme, and dried basil.
5. Cover and cook for another 5-10 minutes, or until the vegetables are tender and the turkey is fully cooked.
6. Serve warm.

Nutrition Info (per serving)
- Calories: 320
- Protein: 25g
- Carbohydrates: 28g
- Fiber: 6g
- Sugars: 6g
- Fat: 12g
- Saturated Fat: 3g
- Sodium: 140mg

Serves
- **4 servings**

Cooking Time
- **Total time: 30 minutes**

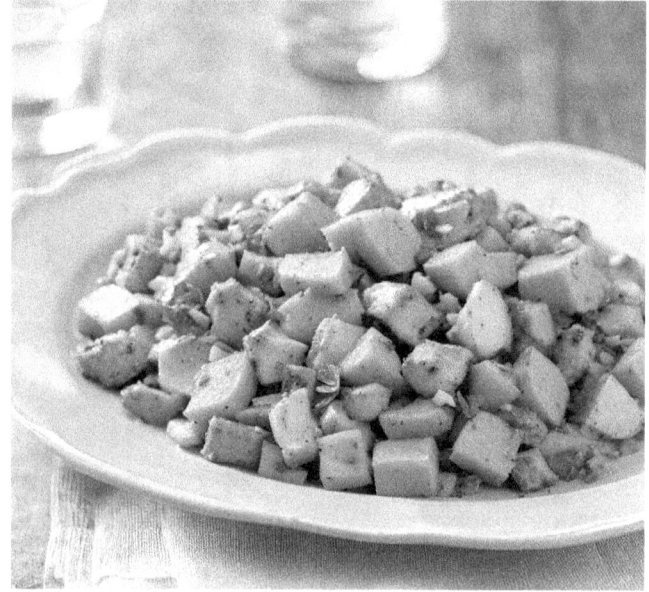

24. Oat-Crusted Turkey Cutlets

Ingredients
- 4 turkey cutlets (about 4 ounces each)
- 1 cup rolled oats, finely ground
- 1/2 cup low-fat milk
- 1 large egg
- 2 tablespoons olive oil
- 1 teaspoon dried oregano
- 1 teaspoon dried basil

Instructions
1. In a shallow bowl, whisk together the low-fat milk and egg.
2. In another shallow bowl, combine the ground oats, dried oregano, and dried basil.
3. Dip each turkey cutlet into the milk mixture, then coat with the oat mixture.
4. Heat the olive oil in a large skillet over medium heat.
5. Cook the turkey cutlets for about 5-6 minutes on each side, or until fully cooked and golden brown.
6. Serve warm.

Nutrition Info (per serving)
- Calories: 280
- Protein: 26g
- Carbohydrates: 18g
- Fiber: 3g
- Sugars: 2g
- Fat: 12g
- Saturated Fat: 2g
- Sodium: 100mg

Serves
- **4 servings**

Cooking Time
- **Total time: 20 minutes**

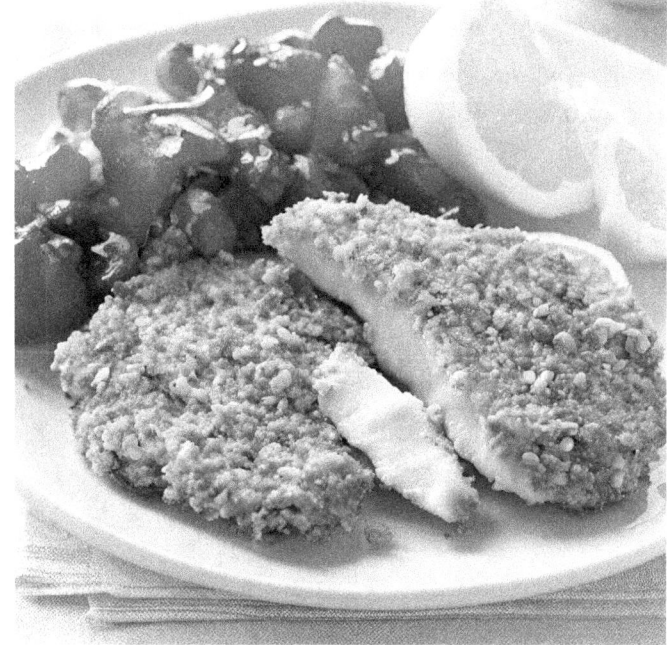

25. Chicken and Vegetable Stir-fry

Ingredients
- 2 boneless, skinless chicken breasts, thinly sliced
- 1 cup zucchini, sliced
- 1 cup carrots, julienned
- 1 cup snap peas
- 2 tablespoons olive oil
- 1 tablespoon low-sodium soy sauce
- 1 teaspoon ground ginger

Instructions
1. Heat 1 tablespoon of olive oil in a large skillet or wok over medium-high heat.
2. Add the sliced chicken and cook until browned, about 5-7 minutes.
3. Remove the chicken from the skillet and set aside.
4. Add the remaining tablespoon of olive oil to the skillet.
5. Add the zucchini, carrots, and snap peas. Stir-fry for 5-7 minutes, or until the vegetables are tender-crisp.
6. Return the chicken to the skillet.
7. Add the low-sodium soy sauce and ground ginger. Stir well to combine and cook for another 2-3 minutes until everything is heated through.
8. Serve warm.

Nutrition Info (per serving)
- Calories: 240
- Protein: 26g
- Carbohydrates: 10g
- Fiber: 3g
- Sugars: 4g
- Fat: 12g
- Saturated Fat: 2g
- Sodium: 200mg

Serves
- 4 servings

Cooking Time
- **Total time: 20 minutes**

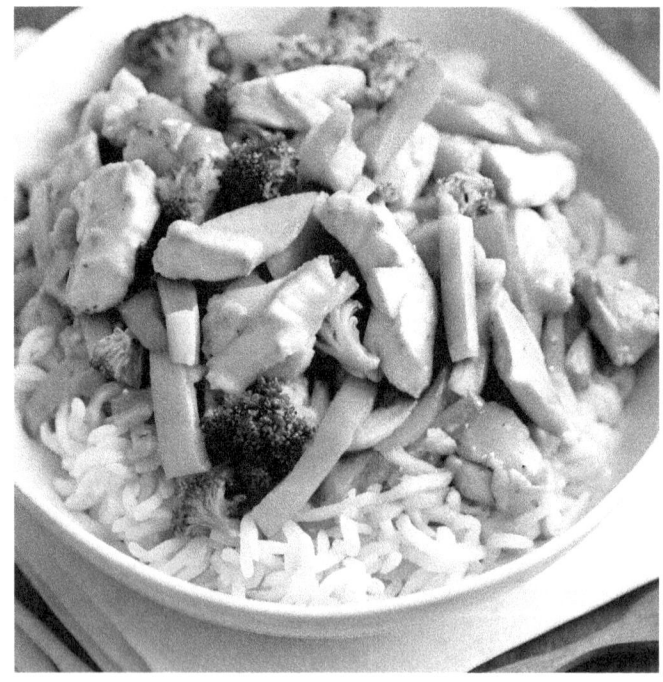

26. Turkey Meatballs

Ingredients
- 1 pound ground turkey
- 1/2 cup rolled oats
- 1/4 cup low-fat milk
- 1 large egg
- 1 teaspoon dried thyme
- 1 teaspoon dried basil
- 1 tablespoon olive oil

Instructions
1. Preheat your oven to 375°F (190°C). Line a baking sheet with parchment paper.
2. In a large bowl, combine the ground turkey, rolled oats, low-fat milk, egg, dried thyme, and dried basil. Mix until well combined.
3. Form the mixture into meatballs, about 1 inch in diameter, and place them on the prepared baking sheet.
4. Heat the olive oil in a skillet over medium heat.
5. Brown the meatballs in the skillet for about 2 minutes on each side.
6. Transfer the browned meatballs to the baking sheet.
7. Bake in the preheated oven for 15-20 minutes, or until the meatballs are fully cooked.
8. Serve warm.

Nutrition Info (per serving)
- Calories: 220
- Protein: 25g
- Carbohydrates: 8g
- Fiber: 2g
- Sugars: 1g
- Fat: 10g
- Saturated Fat: 2g
- Sodium: 100mg

Serves
- 4 servings

Cooking Time
- **Total time: 35 minutes**

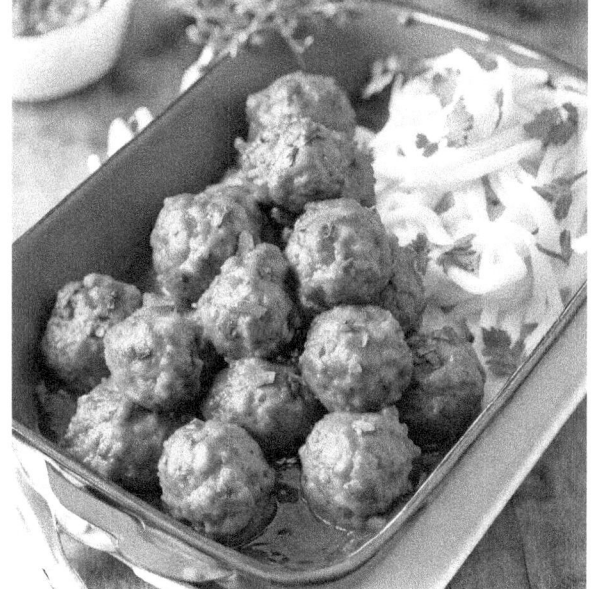

Fish & Seafood Recipes

1. Steamed Cod
Ingredients
- 2 cod fillets (about 4 ounces each)
- 1 tablespoon olive oil
- 1 teaspoon dried thyme
- 1 teaspoon dried parsley
- 1 lemon, sliced (optional)
- Fresh parsley, chopped (for garnish)

Instructions
1. Fill a large pot with 1-2 inches of water and bring to a boil.
2. Place the cod fillets in a steamer basket and brush with olive oil.
3. Sprinkle the dried thyme and dried parsley evenly over the cod fillets.
4. Place the lemon slices (if using) on top of the fillets.
5. Cover and steam the cod for 8-10 minutes, or until the fish is opaque and flakes easily with a fork.
6. Remove the cod from the steamer and place on a serving plate.
7. Garnish with chopped fresh parsley and serve warm.

Nutrition Info (per serving)
- Calories: 150
- Protein: 28g
- Carbohydrates: 1g
- Fiber: 0g
- Sugars: 0g
- Fat: 4g
- Saturated Fat: 1g
- Sodium: 75mg

Serves
- 2 servings

Cooking Time
- Total time: 15 minutes

2. Poached Salmon

Ingredients
- 2 salmon fillets (about 4 ounces each)
- 2 cups low-sodium vegetable broth
- 1 tablespoon olive oil
- 1 teaspoon dried dill
- 1 teaspoon ground ginger
- Fresh dill, chopped (for garnish)

Instructions
1. In a large skillet, bring the vegetable broth to a simmer over medium heat.
2. Add the salmon fillets to the skillet, skin-side down.
3. Sprinkle the dried dill and ground ginger evenly over the salmon fillets.
4. Cover and poach the salmon for 10-12 minutes, or until the fish is opaque and flakes easily with a fork.
5. Carefully remove the salmon from the skillet and place on a serving plate.
6. Drizzle with olive oil and garnish with chopped fresh dill.
7. Serve warm.

Nutrition Info (per serving)
- Calories: 250
- Protein: 22g
- Carbohydrates: 1g
- Fiber: 0g
- Sugars: 0g
- Fat: 17g
- Saturated Fat: 3g
- Sodium: 90mg

Serves
- **2 servings**

Cooking Time
- **Total time: 20 minutes**

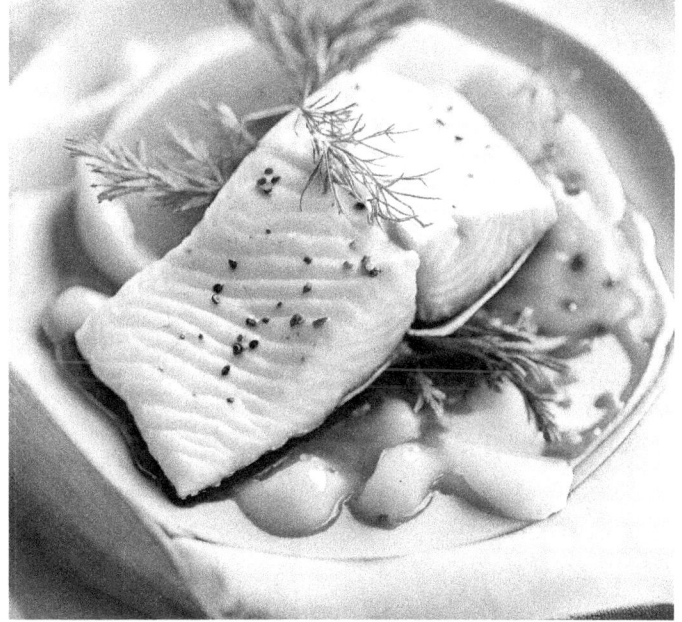

3. Baked Tilapia

Ingredients
- 2 tilapia fillets (about 4 ounces each)
- 1 tablespoon olive oil
- 1 teaspoon dried basil
- 1 teaspoon dried oregano
- 1/4 cup low-fat mozzarella cheese, shredded
- Fresh basil, chopped (for garnish)

Instructions
1. Preheat your oven to 375°F (190°C). Lightly grease a baking dish.
2. Place the tilapia fillets in the baking dish.
3. Brush the fillets with olive oil.
4. Sprinkle the dried basil and dried oregano evenly over the fillets.
5. Sprinkle the shredded mozzarella cheese over the top.
6. Cover with foil and bake for 15 minutes.
7. Remove the foil and bake for an additional 5-10 minutes, or until the fish is opaque and the cheese is melted and golden brown.
8. Remove from the oven and place on a serving plate.
9. Garnish with chopped fresh basil and serve warm.

Nutrition Info (per serving)
- Calories: 220
- Protein: 28g
- Carbohydrates: 2g
- Fiber: 0g
- Sugars: 0g
- Fat: 11g
- Saturated Fat: 3g
- Sodium: 120mg

Serves
- 2 servings

Cooking Time
- **Total time: 25 minutes**

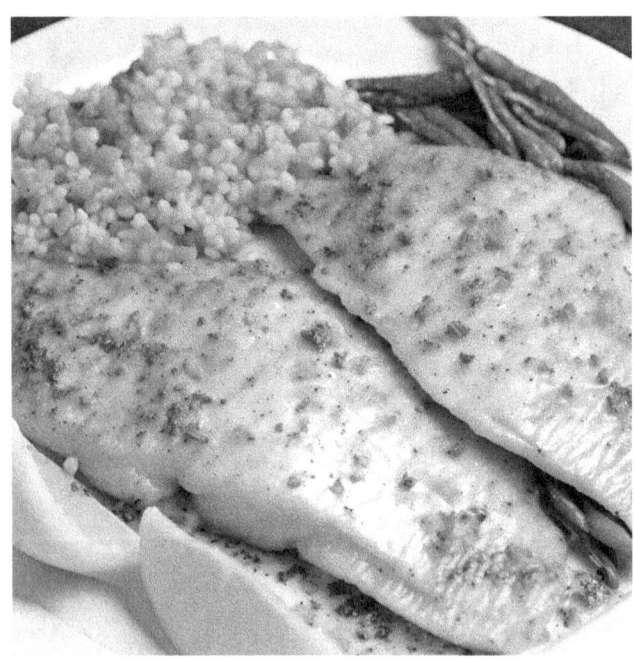

4. Grilled Shrimp

Ingredients
- 1 pound large shrimp, peeled and deveined
- 2 tablespoons olive oil
- 1 teaspoon dried oregano
- 1 teaspoon dried basil
- 1 tablespoon lemon juice (if tolerated)
- Fresh parsley, chopped (for garnish)

Instructions
1. Preheat your grill to medium-high heat.
2. In a bowl, toss the shrimp with olive oil, dried oregano, dried basil, and lemon juice (if tolerated).
3. Thread the shrimp onto skewers.
4. Grill the shrimp for 2-3 minutes on each side, until they are pink and opaque.
5. Remove from the grill and place on a serving plate.
6. Garnish with chopped fresh parsley and serve warm.

Nutrition Info (per serving)
- Calories: 180
- Protein: 24g
- Carbohydrates: 1g
- Fiber: 0g
- Sugars: 0g
- Fat: 8g
- Saturated Fat: 1g
- Sodium: 190mg

Serves
- 4 servings

Cooking Time
- **Total time: 15 minutes**

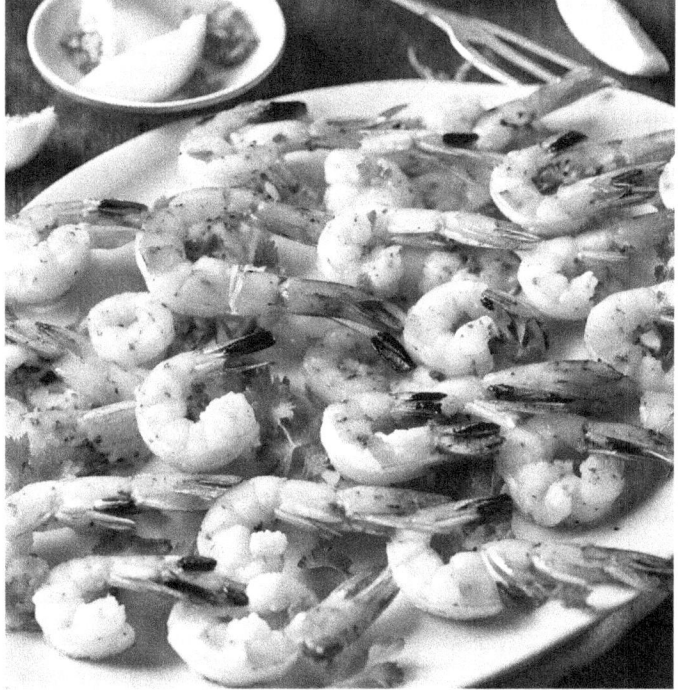

5. Clam Soup

Ingredients
- 1 pound fresh clams, scrubbed clean
- 4 cups low-sodium vegetable broth
- 1 cup diced carrots
- 1 cup diced celery
- 2 tablespoons olive oil
- 1 teaspoon dried thyme
- 1 teaspoon dried parsley

Instructions
1. Heat the olive oil in a large pot over medium heat.
2. Add the diced carrots and celery, and cook for about 5 minutes, until they are tender.
3. Add the low-sodium vegetable broth and bring to a boil.
4. Add the clams and cover the pot.
5. Cook for about 5-7 minutes, or until the clams open. Discard any clams that do not open.
6. Stir in the dried thyme and dried parsley.
7. Serve warm

Nutrition Info (per serving)
- Calories: 180
- Protein: 14g
- Carbohydrates: 10g
- Fiber: 2g
- Sugars: 4g
- Fat: 9g
- Saturated Fat: 1g
- Sodium: 220mg

Serves
- **4 servings**

Cooking Time
- **Total time: 20 minutes**

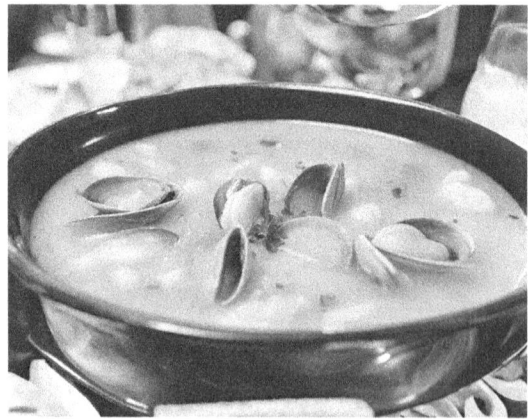

6. Baked Haddock

Ingredients
- 2 haddock fillets (about 4 ounces each)
- 1/4 cup low-fat mozzarella cheese, shredded
- 2 tablespoons olive oil
- 1 teaspoon dried dill
- 1 teaspoon dried parsley
- Lemon wedges (for garnish, if tolerated)

Instructions
1. Preheat your oven to 375°F (190°C). Lightly grease a baking dish.
2. Place the haddock fillets in the baking dish.
3. Brush the fillets with olive oil.
4. Sprinkle the dried dill and dried parsley evenly over the fillets.
5. Top with shredded mozzarella cheese.
6. Cover with foil and bake for 15 minutes.
7. Remove the foil and bake for an additional 5-10 minutes, or until the fish is opaque and the cheese is melted and golden brown.
8. Serve warm, with lemon wedges on the side (if tolerated).

Nutrition Info (per serving)
- Calories: 220
- Protein: 28g
- Carbohydrates: 1g
- Fiber: 0g
- Sugars: 0g
- Fat: 12g
- Saturated Fat: 3g
- Sodium: 160mg

Serves
- 2 servings

Cooking Time
- **Total time: 25 minutes**

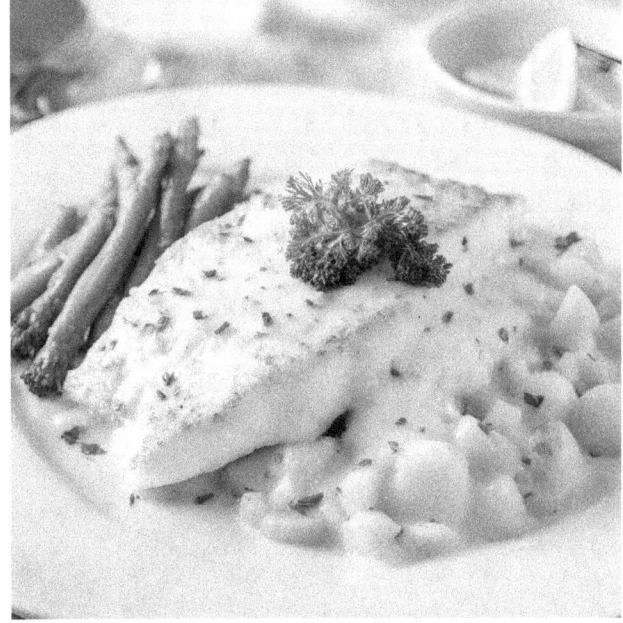

7. Ginger Shrimp Stir Fry

Ingredients
- 1 pound large shrimp, peeled and deveined
- 1 cup snap peas
- 1 cup sliced carrots
- 1 cup sliced zucchini
- 2 tablespoons olive oil
- 1 tablespoon grated fresh ginger
- 2 tablespoons low-sodium soy sauce

Instructions
1. Heat 1 tablespoon of olive oil in a large skillet or wok over medium-high heat.
2. Add the shrimp and cook until pink and opaque, about 2-3 minutes. Remove from the skillet and set aside.
3. Add the remaining tablespoon of olive oil to the skillet.
4. Add the snap peas, carrots, zucchini, and grated ginger. Stir-fry for 5-7 minutes, or until the vegetables are tender-crisp.
5. Return the shrimp to the skillet.
6. Add the low-sodium soy sauce and stir well to combine. Cook for another 2-3 minutes until everything is heated through.
7. Serve warm.

Nutrition Info (per serving)
- Calories: 220
- Protein: 24g
- Carbohydrates: 8g
- Fiber: 2g
- Sugars: 3g
- Fat: 10g
- Saturated Fat: 1.5g
- Sodium: 320mg

Serves
- 4 servings

Cooking Time
- **Total time: 20 minutes**

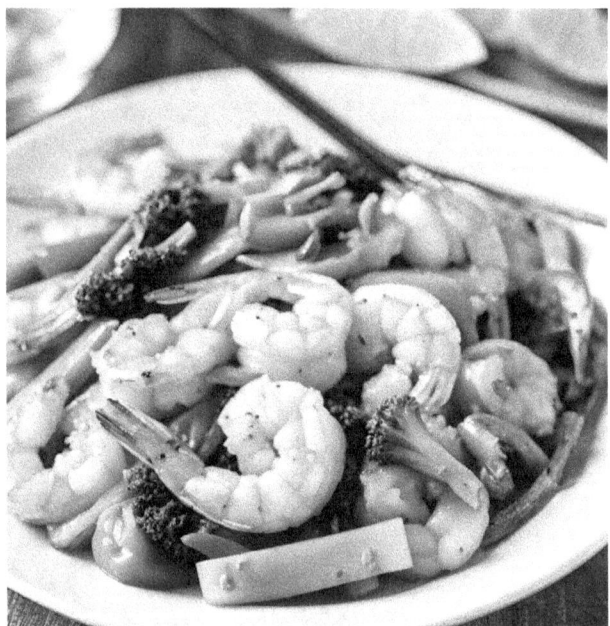

8. Oven-Poached Flounder

Ingredients
- 2 flounder fillets (about 4 ounces each)
- 1 cup low-sodium vegetable broth
- 1 tablespoon olive oil
- 1 teaspoon dried thyme
- 1 teaspoon dried basil
- Lemon wedges (for garnish, if tolerated)

Instructions
1. Preheat your oven to 375°F (190°C). Lightly grease a baking dish.
2. Place the flounder fillets in the baking dish.
3. Pour the low-sodium vegetable broth over the fillets.
4. Drizzle with olive oil and sprinkle with dried thyme and dried basil.
5. Cover with foil and bake for 15-20 minutes, or until the fish is opaque and flakes easily with a fork.
6. Remove from the oven and place on a serving plate.
7. Serve warm with lemon wedges on the side (if tolerated).

Nutrition Info (per serving)
- Calories: 180
- Protein: 26g
- Carbohydrates: 2g
- Fiber: 0g
- Sugars: 0g
- Fat: 7g
- Saturated Fat: 1g
- Sodium: 140mg

Serves
- 2 servings

Cooking Time
- **Total time: 25 minutes**

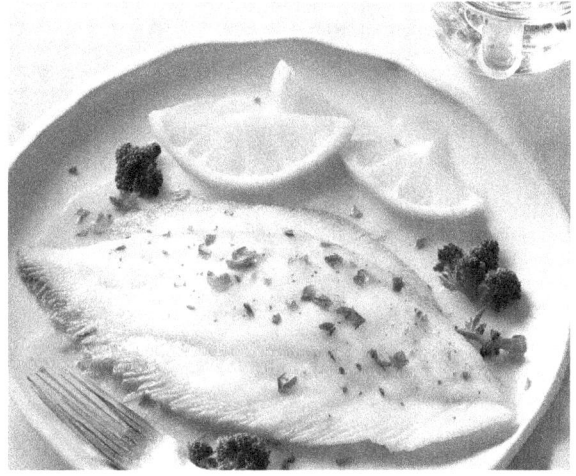

9. Salmon and Potato Bake

Ingredients
- 2 salmon fillets (about 4 ounces each)
- 2 medium potatoes, peeled and thinly sliced
- 1 cup low-fat milk
- 1 tablespoon olive oil
- 1 teaspoon dried dill
- 1 teaspoon dried thyme
- 1/4 cup low-fat mozzarella cheese, shredded

Instructions
1. Preheat your oven to 375°F (190°C). Lightly grease a baking dish.
2. Arrange the thinly sliced potatoes in the baking dish.
3. Place the salmon fillets on top of the potatoes.
4. In a small bowl, mix together the low-fat milk, olive oil, dried dill, and dried thyme.
5. Pour the mixture over the salmon and potatoes.
6. Sprinkle the shredded mozzarella cheese over the top.
7. Cover with foil and bake for 25 minutes.
8. Remove the foil and bake for an additional 10-15 minutes, or until the salmon is fully cooked and the potatoes are tender.
9. Serve warm.

Nutrition Info (per serving)
- Calories: 320
- Protein: 28g
- Carbohydrates: 20g
- Fiber: 3g
- Sugars: 3g
- Fat: 14g
- Saturated Fat: 4g
- Sodium: 150mg

Serves
- **2 servings**

Cooking Time
- **Total time: 40 minutes**

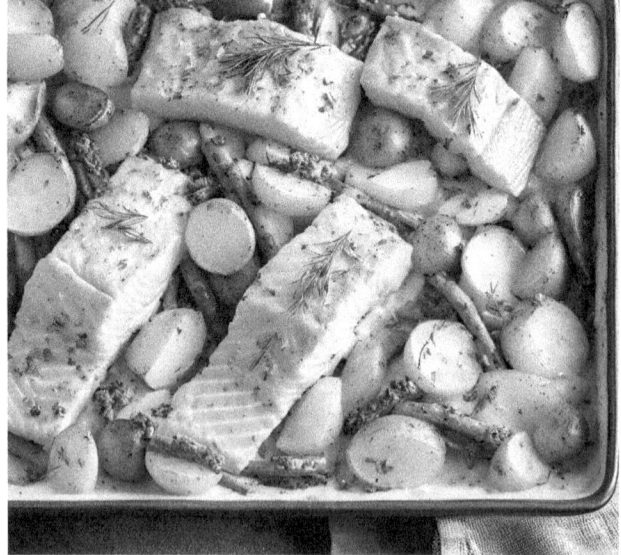

10. Shrimp and Rice Pilaf

Ingredients
- 1 pound large shrimp, peeled and deveined
- 1 cup basmati rice
- 2 cups low-sodium chicken broth
- 1 cup peas
- 1 tablespoon olive oil
- 1 teaspoon dried basil
- 1 teaspoon dried thyme

Instructions
1. Heat the olive oil in a large pot over medium heat.
2. Add the basmati rice and cook for 2 minutes, stirring frequently.
3. Pour in the chicken broth and bring to a boil.
4. Reduce the heat, cover, and simmer for 15 minutes.
5. Stir in the peas and shrimp, and sprinkle with dried basil and dried thyme.
6. Cover and cook for an additional 5-7 minutes, or until the shrimp are pink and opaque and the rice is tender.
7. Serve warm.

Nutrition Info (per serving)
- Calories: 320
- Protein: 28g
- Carbohydrates: 40g
- Fiber: 4g
- Sugars: 3g
- Fat: 7g
- Saturated Fat: 1g
- Sodium: 210mg

Serves
- 4 servings

Cooking Time
- **Total time: 25 minutes**

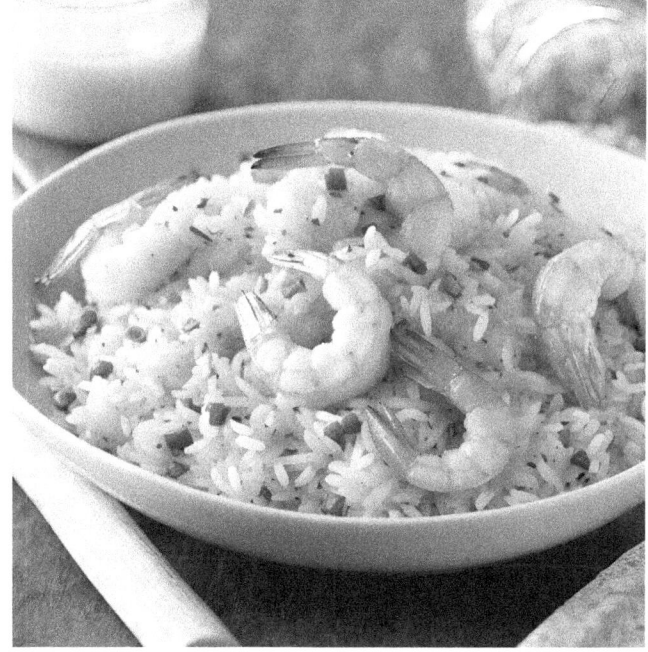

11. Crab Stuffed Mushrooms

Ingredients
- 12 large white mushrooms, stems removed
- 1 cup lump crab meat
- 1/4 cup low-fat cream cheese
- 1 tablespoon chopped fresh parsley
- 1 teaspoon dried dill
- 2 tablespoons olive oil

Instructions
1. Preheat your oven to 375°F (190°C). Lightly grease a baking sheet.
2. In a bowl, combine the crab meat, low-fat cream cheese, chopped parsley, and dried dill.
3. Fill each mushroom cap with the crab mixture.
4. Arrange the stuffed mushrooms on the prepared baking sheet.
5. Drizzle the olive oil over the mushrooms.
6. Bake for 15-20 minutes, or until the mushrooms are tender and the filling is heated through.
7. Serve warm.

Nutrition Info (per serving)
- Calories: 150
- Protein: 12g
- Carbohydrates: 4g
- Fiber: 1g
- Sugars: 2g
- Fat: 10g
- Saturated Fat: 3g
- Sodium: 180mg

Serves
- 4 servings

Cooking Time
- **Total time: 25 minutes**

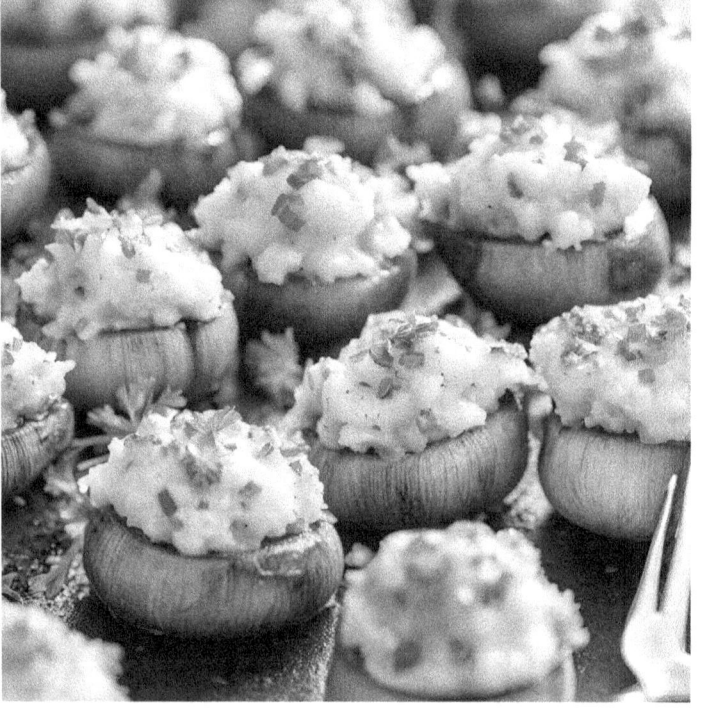

12. Scallops with Peas

Ingredients
- 1 pound sea scallops
- 1 cup peas
- 2 tablespoons olive oil
- 1 teaspoon dried thyme
- 1 teaspoon ground ginger
- Fresh parsley, chopped (for garnish)

Instructions
1. Heat 1 tablespoon of olive oil in a large skillet over medium-high heat.
2. Add the scallops and cook for 2-3 minutes on each side, until they are golden brown and opaque. Remove from the skillet and set aside.
3. Add the remaining tablespoon of olive oil to the skillet.
4. Add the peas and cook for 3-4 minutes, until they are tender.
5. Return the scallops to the skillet.
6. Sprinkle with dried thyme and ground ginger. Stir to combine and cook for another 1-2 minutes until everything is heated through.
7. Serve warm, garnished with chopped fresh parsley.

Nutrition Info (per serving)
- Calories: 210
- Protein: 24g
- Carbohydrates: 10g
- Fiber: 3g
- Sugars: 3g
- Fat: 8g
- Saturated Fat: 1.5g
- Sodium: 210mg

Serves
- 4 servings

Cooking Time
- **Total time: 15 minutes**

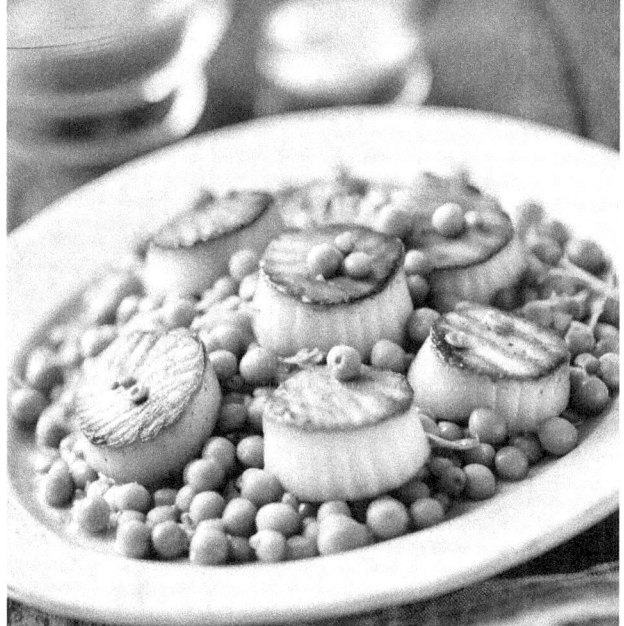

13. Mackerel in Oatmeal

Ingredients
- 2 mackerel fillets
- 1 cup rolled oats
- 1/2 cup low-fat milk
- 1 tablespoon olive oil
- 1 teaspoon dried thyme
- 1 teaspoon dried parsley

Instructions
1. Preheat your oven to 375°F (190°C). Lightly grease a baking dish.
2. In a shallow bowl, soak the rolled oats in the low-fat milk for 5 minutes.
3. Coat each mackerel fillet with the soaked oats.
4. Place the coated fillets in the baking dish.
5. Drizzle with olive oil and sprinkle with dried thyme and dried parsley.
6. Bake for 20-25 minutes, or until the fish is cooked through and the oats are golden brown.
7. Serve warm.

Nutrition Info (per serving)
- Calories: 280
- Protein: 20g
- Carbohydrates: 18g
- Fiber: 4g
- Sugars: 2g
- Fat: 14g
- Saturated Fat: 3g
- Sodium: 120mg

Serves
- 2 servings

Cooking Time
- **Total time: 30 minutes**

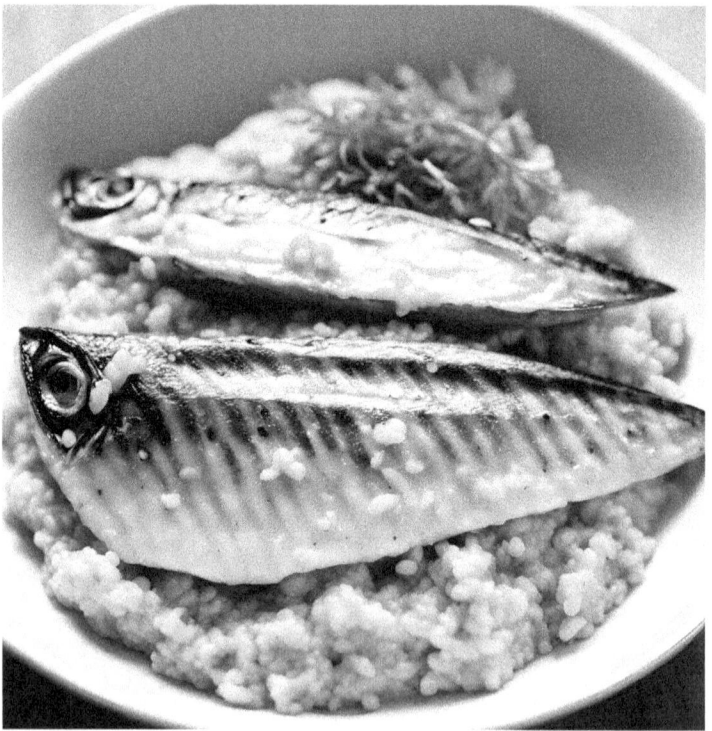

14. Lobster and Rice

Ingredients
- 2 lobster tails
- 1 cup basmati rice
- 2 cups low-sodium chicken broth
- 1 cup peas
- 1 tablespoon olive oil
- 1 teaspoon dried basil
- 1 teaspoon dried oregano

Instructions
1. Preheat your oven to 375°F (190°C).
2. In a large pot, bring the low-sodium chicken broth to a boil.
3. Add the basmati rice, reduce the heat, cover, and simmer for 15 minutes.
4. Meanwhile, steam the lobster tails for 8-10 minutes, or until the shells are bright red and the meat is opaque.
5. Remove the lobster meat from the shells and chop into bite-sized pieces.
6. In a large skillet, heat the olive oil over medium heat.
7. Add the peas, dried basil, and dried oregano. Cook for 5 minutes, stirring occasionally.
8. Add the cooked rice and lobster meat to the skillet. Stir to combine and cook for an additional 3-5 minutes until heated through.
9. Serve warm.

Nutrition Info (per serving)
- Calories: 320
- Protein: 28g
- Carbohydrates: 30g
- Fiber: 3g
- Sugars: 2g
- Fat: 10g
- Saturated Fat: 2g
- Sodium: 240mg

Serves
- 2 servings

Cooking Time
- **Total time: 30 minutes**

15. Salmon Salad

Ingredients
- 2 salmon fillets (about 4 ounces each), grilled and flaked
- 4 cups mixed greens (spinach, arugula, lettuce)
- 1/2 cup cucumber, diced
- 1/2 cup cherry tomatoes, halved (if tolerated)
- 1/4 cup low-fat feta cheese, crumbled
- 2 tablespoons olive oil
- 1 tablespoon lemon juice (if tolerated)
- 1 teaspoon dried dill

Instructions
1. In a large salad bowl, combine the mixed greens, diced cucumber, and cherry tomatoes.
2. Add the flaked grilled salmon and crumbled feta cheese on top.
3. In a small bowl, whisk together the olive oil, lemon juice, and dried dill.
4. Drizzle the dressing over the salad and toss gently to combine.
5. Serve immediately.

Nutrition Info (per serving)
- Calories: 300
- Protein: 26g
- Carbohydrates: 8g
- Fiber: 3g
- Sugars: 4g
- Fat: 18g
- Saturated Fat: 4g
- Sodium: 220mg

Serves
- 2 servings

Cooking Time
- **Total time: 15 minutes (plus grilling time for the salmon)**

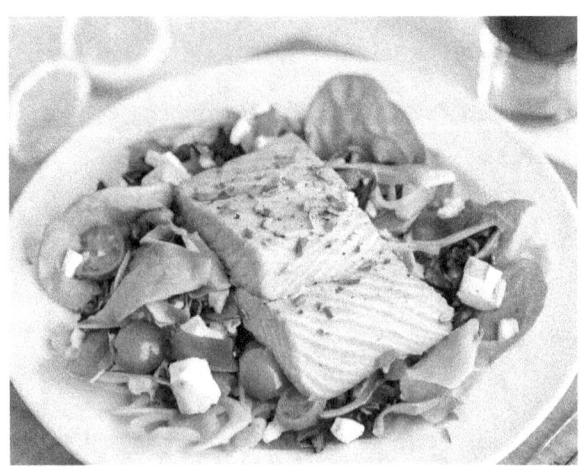

16. Grilled Sole

Ingredients
- 2 sole fillets (about 4 ounces each)
- 2 tablespoons olive oil
- 1 teaspoon dried oregano
- 1 teaspoon dried basil
- Lemon wedges (for garnish, if tolerated)

Instructions
1. Preheat your grill to medium-high heat.
2. Brush the sole fillets with olive oil.
3. Sprinkle the dried oregano and dried basil evenly over the fillets.
4. Grill the sole for 2-3 minutes on each side, or until the fish is opaque and flakes easily with a fork.
5. Remove from the grill and place on a serving plate.
6. Serve warm with lemon wedges on the side (if tolerated).

Nutrition Info (per serving)
- Calories: 180
- Protein: 24g
- Carbohydrates: 1g
- Fiber: 0g
- Sugars: 0g
- Fat: 8g
- Saturated Fat: 1g
- Sodium: 140mg

Serves
- 2 servings

Cooking Time
- **Total time: 10 minutes**

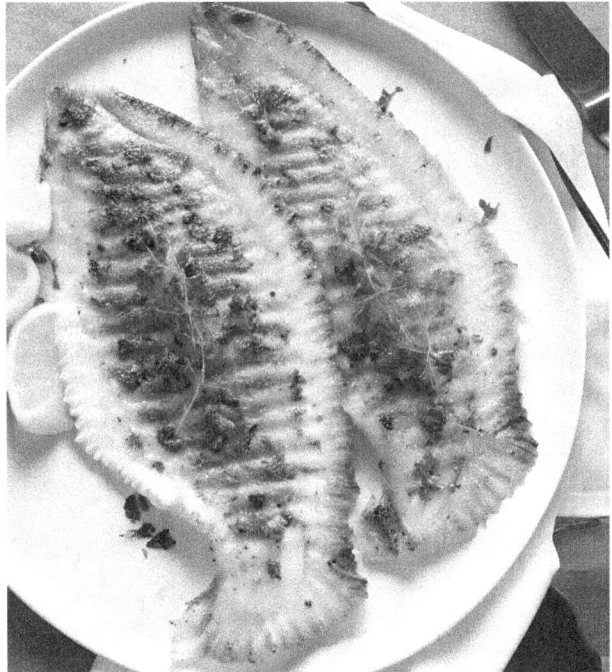

17. Clam and Potato Casserole

Ingredients

- 1 pound fresh clams, scrubbed clean
- 2 medium potatoes, peeled and diced
- 1 cup diced carrots
- 1 cup diced celery
- 2 tablespoons olive oil
- 2 cups low-sodium vegetable broth
- 1 teaspoon dried thyme
- 1 teaspoon dried parsley

Instructions

1. Preheat your oven to 375°F (190°C).
2. In a large pot, heat the olive oil over medium heat. Add the diced carrots and celery, and cook for about 5 minutes until tender.
3. Add the diced potatoes and cook for another 5 minutes.
4. Pour in the vegetable broth, add the dried thyme and dried parsley, and bring to a boil.
5. Add the clams, cover the pot, and cook until the clams open, about 5-7 minutes. Discard any clams that do not open.
6. Transfer the mixture to a baking dish and bake for 15 minutes.
7. Serve warm.

Nutrition Info (per serving)

- Calories: 220
- Protein: 12g
- Carbohydrates: 28g
- Fiber: 4g
- Sugars: 3g
- Fat: 8g
- Saturated Fat: 1g
- Sodium: 200mg

Serves

- 4 servings

Cooking Time

- **Total time: 40 minutes**

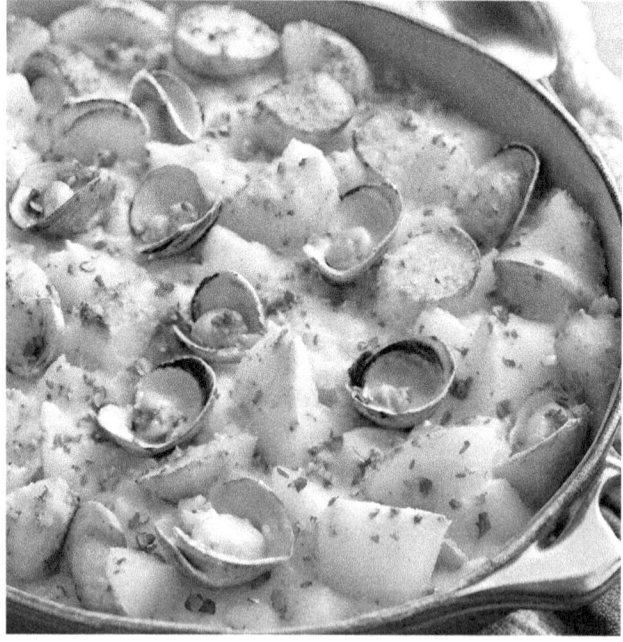

18. Baked Sea Bass

Ingredients
- 2 sea bass fillets (about 4 ounces each)
- 2 tablespoons olive oil
- 1 teaspoon dried basil
- 1 teaspoon dried oregano
- Lemon wedges (for garnish, if tolerated)

Instructions
1. Preheat your oven to 375°F (190°C). Lightly grease a baking dish.
2. Brush the sea bass fillets with olive oil.
3. Sprinkle the dried basil and dried oregano evenly over the fillets.
4. Place the fillets in the baking dish and cover with foil.
5. Bake for 20-25 minutes, or until the fish is opaque and flakes easily with a fork.
6. Serve warm with lemon wedges on the side (if tolerated).

Nutrition Info (per serving)
- Calories: 180
- Protein: 24g
- Carbohydrates: 1g
- Fiber: 0g
- Sugars: 0g
- Fat: 8g
- Saturated Fat: 1g
- Sodium: 140mg

Serves
- 2 servings

Cooking Time
- **Total time: 25 minutes**

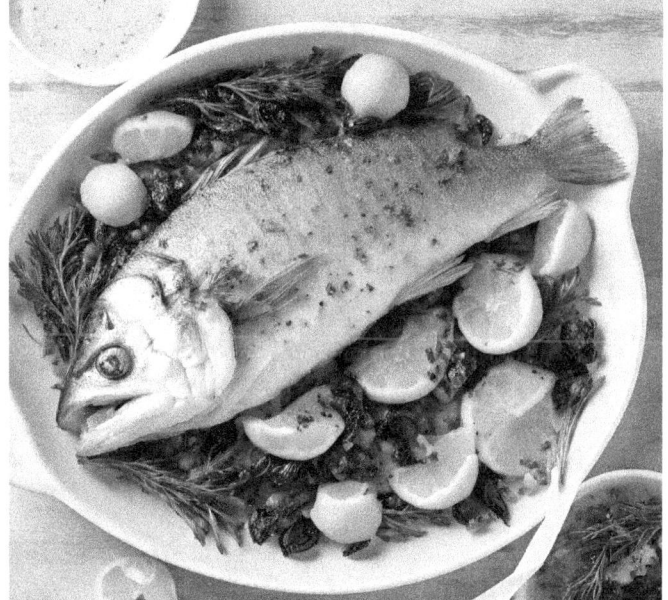

19. Poached Pear and Salmon

Ingredients
- 2 salmon fillets (about 4 ounces each)
- 2 ripe pears, peeled, cored, and sliced
- 2 cups low-sodium vegetable broth
- 1 tablespoon olive oil
- 1 teaspoon ground ginger
- Fresh parsley, chopped (for garnish)

Instructions
1. In a large skillet, bring the vegetable broth to a simmer over medium heat.
2. Add the salmon fillets and poach for 8-10 minutes, or until the fish is opaque and flakes easily with a fork.
3. In a separate skillet, heat the olive oil over medium heat.
4. Add the pear slices and ground ginger, and cook for 5-7 minutes, or until the pears are tender.
5. Serve the poached salmon with the gingered pears on the side, garnished with chopped parsley.

Nutrition Info (per serving)
- Calories: 280
- Protein: 22g
- Carbohydrates: 20g
- Fiber: 4g
- Sugars: 12g
- Fat: 12g
- Saturated Fat: 2g
- Sodium: 140mg

Serves
- 2 servings

Cooking Time
- **Total time: 20 minutes**

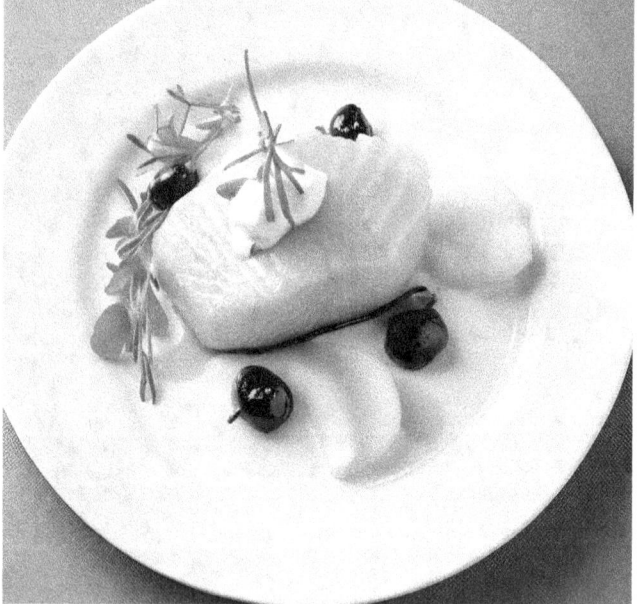

20. Scallop Soup

Ingredients

- 1 pound sea scallops
- 4 cups low-sodium vegetable broth
- 1 cup diced carrots
- 1 cup diced celery
- 2 tablespoons olive oil
- 1 teaspoon dried thyme
- 1 teaspoon dried dill

Instructions

1. In a large pot, heat the olive oil over medium heat.
2. Add the diced carrots and celery, and cook for about 5 minutes until tender.
3. Pour in the vegetable broth and bring to a boil.
4. Add the scallops and reduce the heat to a simmer. Cook for 5-7 minutes, or until the scallops are opaque and cooked through.
5. Stir in the dried thyme and dried dill.
6. Serve warm.

Nutrition Info (per serving)

- Calories: 220
- Protein: 20g
- Carbohydrates: 12g
- Fiber: 2g
- Sugars: 4g
- Fat: 10g
- Saturated Fat: 1.5g
- Sodium: 160mg

Serves

- 4 servings

Cooking Time

- **Total time: 20 minutes**

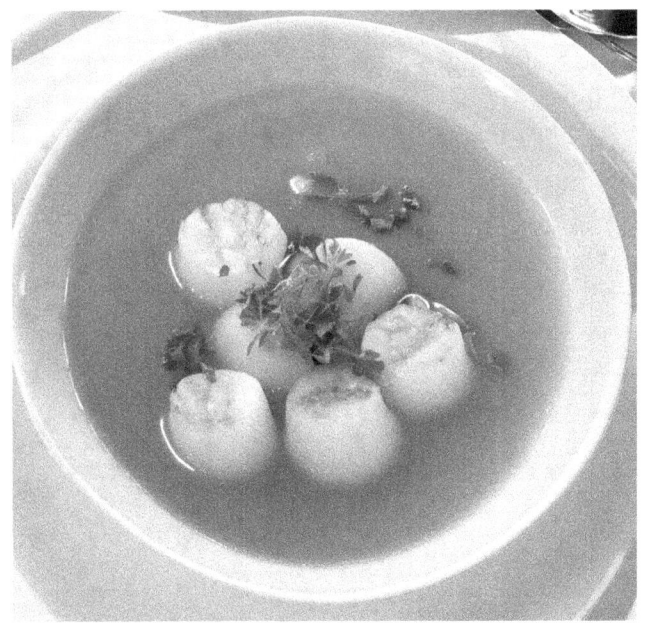

21. Halibut and Zucchini

Ingredients

- 2 halibut fillets (about 4 ounces each)
- 2 medium zucchinis, sliced
- 2 tablespoons olive oil
- 1 teaspoon dried thyme
- 1 teaspoon dried basil
- Fresh parsley, chopped (for garnish)

Instructions

1. Preheat your oven to 375°F (190°C). Lightly grease a baking dish.
2. Arrange the zucchini slices in the baking dish.
3. Place the halibut fillets on top of the zucchini.
4. Drizzle the olive oil over the halibut and zucchini.
5. Sprinkle the dried thyme and dried basil evenly over the halibut and zucchini.
6. Cover with foil and bake for 20-25 minutes, or until the fish is opaque and flakes easily with a fork.
7. Remove from the oven and place on a serving plate.
8. Garnish with chopped fresh parsley and serve warm.

Nutrition Info (per serving)

- Calories: 220
- Protein: 26g
- Carbohydrates: 5g
- Fiber: 2g
- Sugars: 3g
- Fat: 10g
- Saturated Fat: 2g
- Sodium: 120mg

Serves

- 2 servings

Cooking Time

- **Total time: 25 minutes**

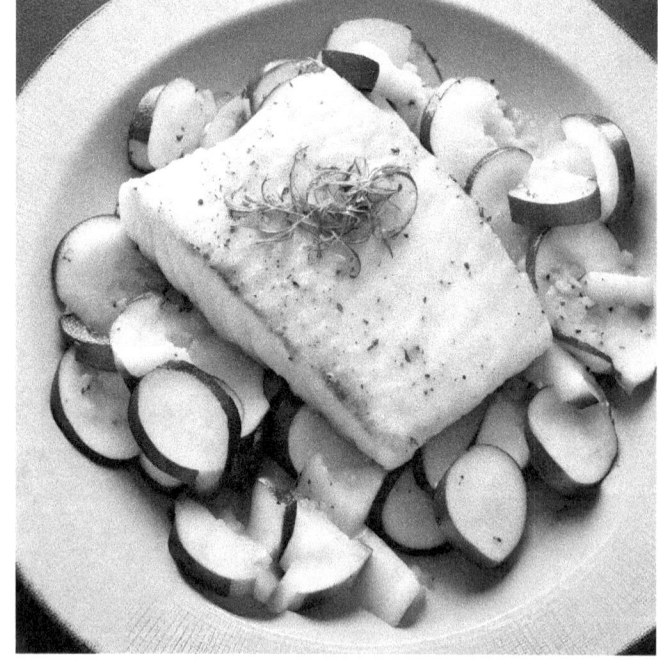

22. Cod and Asparagus Bake

Ingredients
- 2 cod fillets (about 4 ounces each)
- 1 bunch asparagus, trimmed and cut into 2-inch pieces
- 2 tablespoons olive oil
- 1 teaspoon dried dill
- 1 teaspoon dried oregano
- Lemon wedges (for garnish, if tolerated)

Instructions
1. Preheat your oven to 375°F (190°C). Lightly grease a baking dish.
2. Arrange the asparagus pieces in the baking dish.
3. Place the cod fillets on top of the asparagus.
4. Drizzle the olive oil over the cod and asparagus.
5. Sprinkle the dried dill and dried oregano evenly over the cod and asparagus.
6. Cover with foil and bake for 20-25 minutes, or until the fish is opaque and flakes easily with a fork.
7. Remove from the oven and place on a serving plate.
8. Serve warm with lemon wedges on the side (if tolerated).

Nutrition Info (per serving)
- Calories: 210
- Protein: 24g
- Carbohydrates: 5g
- Fiber: 2g
- Sugars: 2g
- Fat: 10g
- Saturated Fat: 2g
- Sodium: 130mg

Serves
- 2 servings

Cooking Time
- **Total time: 25 minutes**

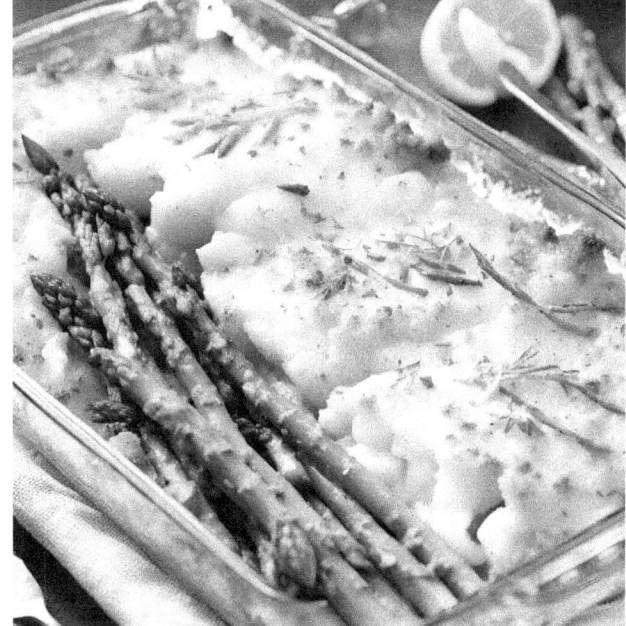

23. Tilapia with Minted Peas
Ingredients
- 2 tilapia fillets (about 4 ounces each)
- 1 cup peas
- 2 tablespoons olive oil
- 1 teaspoon dried mint
- 1 teaspoon dried basil
- Fresh mint leaves, chopped (for garnish)

Instructions
1. Preheat your oven to 375°F (190°C). Lightly grease a baking dish.
2. Place the tilapia fillets in the baking dish.
3. Drizzle the olive oil over the tilapia.
4. Sprinkle the dried mint and dried basil evenly over the tilapia.
5. Bake for 15-20 minutes, or until the fish is opaque and flakes easily with a fork.
6. While the fish is baking, steam the peas for 5-7 minutes, or until tender.
7. Serve the baked tilapia with the steamed peas on the side.
8. Garnish with chopped fresh mint leaves and serve warm.

Nutrition Info (per serving)
- Calories: 220
- Protein: 24g
- Carbohydrates: 10g
- Fiber: 4g
- Sugars: 3g
- Fat: 10g
- Saturated Fat: 2g
- Sodium: 120mg

Serves
- 2 servings

Cooking Time
- **Total time: 20 minutes**

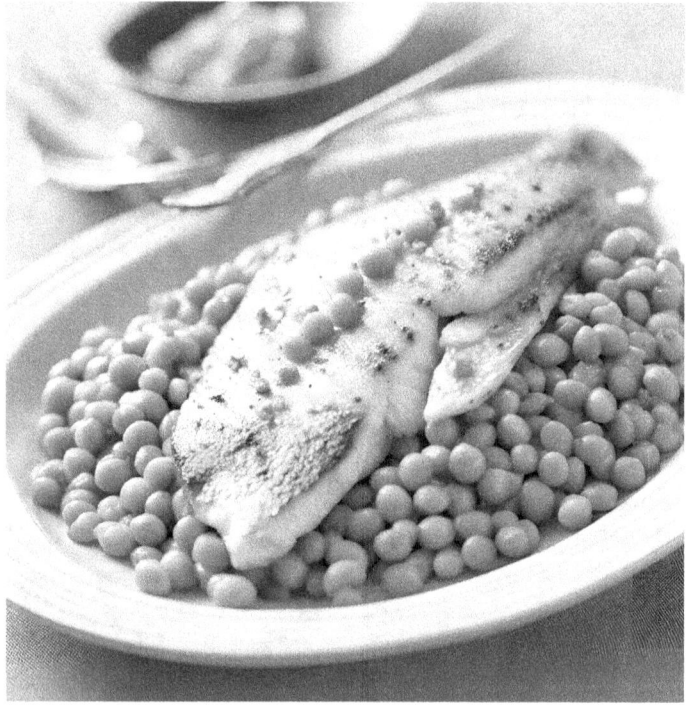

24. Crab and Spinach Noodles

Ingredients
- 8 ounces whole wheat noodles
- 1 cup lump crab meat
- 2 cups fresh spinach leaves
- 1 tablespoon olive oil
- 1/4 cup low-fat cream cheese
- 1 teaspoon dried dill
- 1 teaspoon dried thyme

Instructions
1. Cook the whole wheat noodles according to package instructions. Drain and set aside.
2. In a large skillet, heat the olive oil over medium heat.
3. Add the fresh spinach leaves and cook until wilted, about 3-4 minutes.
4. Add the crab meat, low-fat cream cheese, dried dill, and dried thyme. Stir to combine and cook for another 2-3 minutes until heated through.
5. Toss the cooked noodles with the crab and spinach mixture.
6. Serve warm.

Nutrition Info (per serving)
- Calories: 320
- Protein: 20g
- Carbohydrates: 45g
- Fiber: 6g
- Sugars: 3g
- Fat: 10g
- Saturated Fat: 3g
- Sodium: 160mg

Serves
- 4 servings

Cooking Time
- **Total time: 20 minutes**

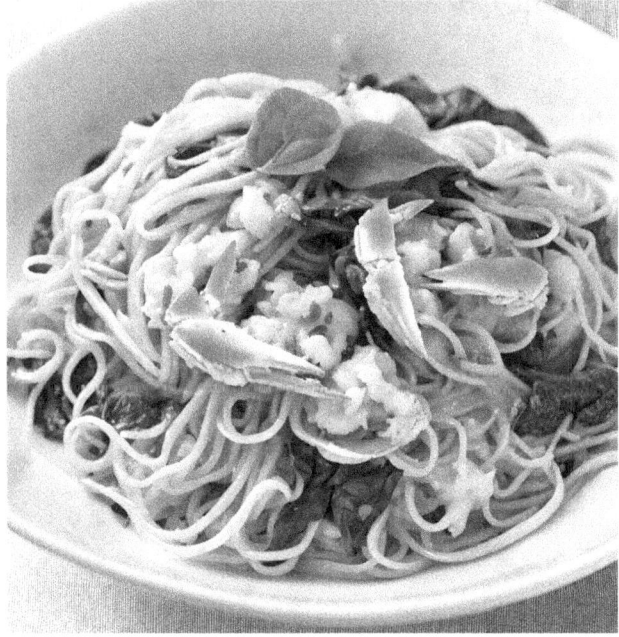

25. Scallops with Parsnip Puree

Ingredients
- 1 pound sea scallops
- 4 medium parsnips, peeled and chopped
- 2 tablespoons olive oil
- 1/2 cup low-fat milk
- 1 teaspoon dried thyme
- Fresh parsley, chopped (for garnish)

Instructions
1. In a large pot, bring the chopped parsnips to a boil in salted water. Cook until tender, about 15 minutes.
2. Drain the parsnips and return them to the pot. Add the low-fat milk and mash until smooth.
3. In a large skillet, heat 1 tablespoon of olive oil over medium-high heat.
4. Add the scallops and cook for 2-3 minutes on each side, until they are golden brown and opaque. Remove from the skillet and set aside.
5. Serve the seared scallops on top of the parsnip puree.
6. Drizzle with the remaining tablespoon of olive oil and garnish with chopped fresh parsley.
7. Serve warm.

Nutrition Info (per serving)
- Calories: 250
- Protein: 24g
- Carbohydrates: 18g
- Fiber: 5g
- Sugars: 6g
- Fat: 10g
- Saturated Fat: 2g
- Sodium: 180mg

Serves
- 4 servings

Cooking Time
- Total time: 25 minutes

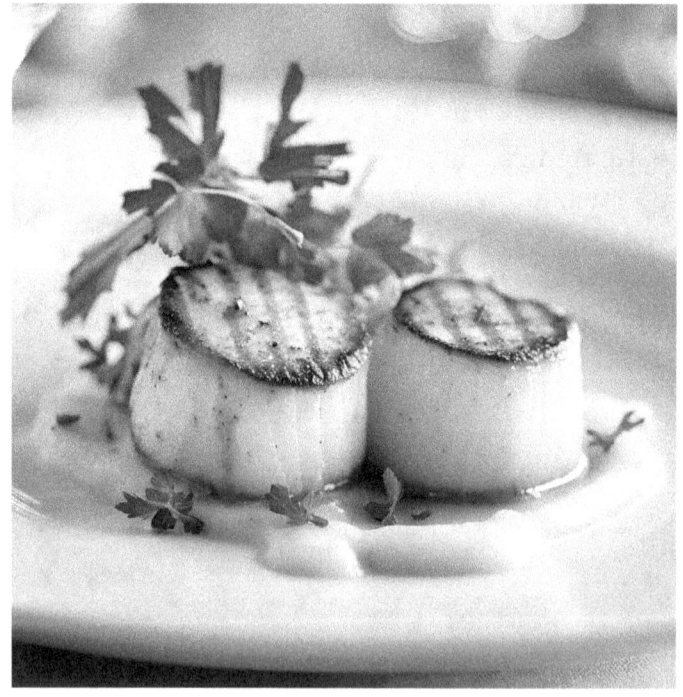

Vegetables

1. Vegetable Stew
Ingredients
- 2 medium potatoes, peeled and diced
- 2 carrots, sliced
- 1 zucchini, diced
- 1 cup green beans, trimmed and cut into 1-inch pieces
- 4 cups low-sodium vegetable broth
- 2 tablespoons olive oil
- 1 teaspoon dried thyme
- 1 teaspoon dried basil

Instructions
1. In a large pot, heat the olive oil over medium heat.
2. Add the diced potatoes, carrots, zucchini, and green beans. Cook for about 5 minutes, stirring occasionally.
3. Pour in the vegetable broth and bring to a boil.
4. Add the dried thyme and dried basil.
5. Reduce the heat, cover, and simmer for 20-25 minutes, or until the vegetables are tender.
6. Serve warm.

Nutrition Info (per serving)
- Calories: 160
- Protein: 4g
- Carbohydrates: 30g
- Fiber: 6g
- Sugars: 6g
- Fat: 5g
- Saturated Fat: 1g
- Sodium: 180mg

Serves
- 4 servings

Cooking Time
- **Total time: 35 minutes**

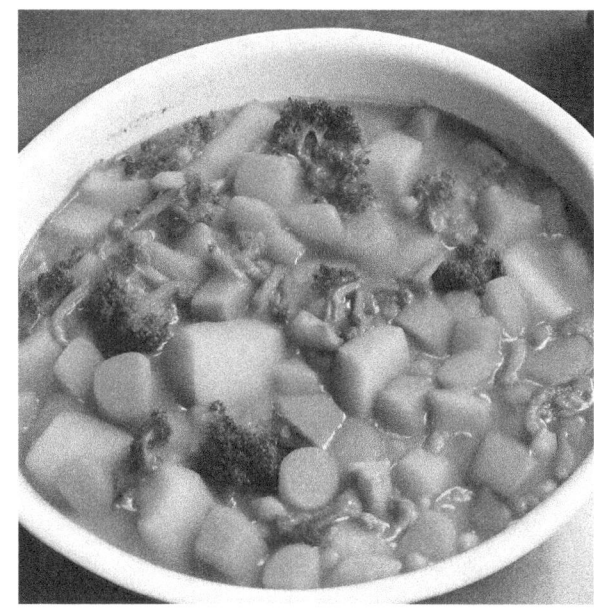

2. Pumpkin and Carrot Bake

Ingredients
- 2 cups pumpkin, peeled and diced
- 2 carrots, peeled and sliced
- 2 tablespoons olive oil
- 1 teaspoon dried rosemary
- 1 teaspoon dried thyme

Instructions
1. Preheat your oven to 375°F (190°C). Lightly grease a baking dish.
2. In a bowl, toss the pumpkin and carrot pieces with olive oil, dried rosemary, and dried thyme.
3. Spread the mixture evenly in the baking dish.
4. Bake for 25-30 minutes, or until the vegetables are tender and slightly caramelized.
5. Serve warm.

Nutrition Info (per serving)
- Calories: 120
- Protein: 2g
- Carbohydrates: 20g
- Fiber: 4g
- Sugars: 8g
- Fat: 5g
- Saturated Fat: 1g
- Sodium: 40mg

Serves
- 4 servings

Cooking Time
- **Total time: 30 minutes**

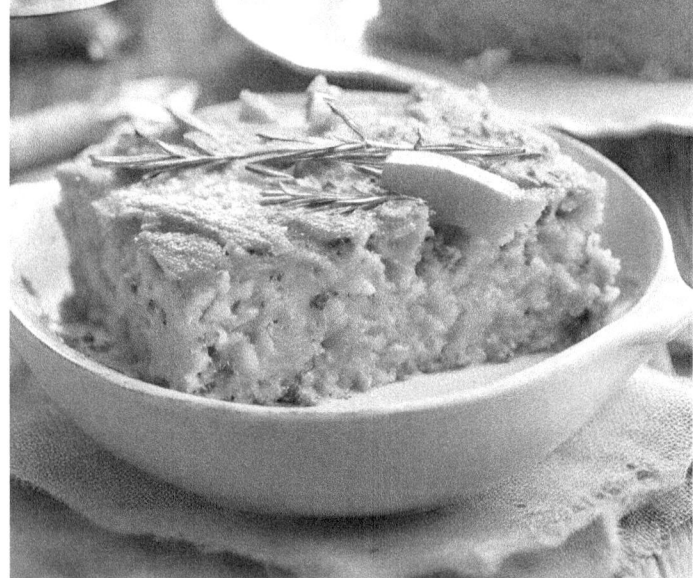

3. Herbed Potato Salad

Ingredients
- 4 medium potatoes, peeled and diced
- 1/4 cup low-fat plain yogurt
- 2 tablespoons olive oil
- 1 tablespoon fresh dill, chopped
- 1 tablespoon fresh parsley, chopped
- 1 teaspoon dried basil

Instructions
1. Boil the diced potatoes in salted water until tender, about 10-15 minutes. Drain and let cool.
2. In a large bowl, combine the cooked potatoes, yogurt, olive oil, fresh dill, fresh parsley, and dried basil.
3. Mix until the potatoes are well coated.
4. Serve chilled or at room temperature.

Nutrition Info (per serving)
- Calories: 180
- Protein: 3g
- Carbohydrates: 30g
- Fiber: 3g
- Sugars: 3g
- Fat: 7g
- Saturated Fat: 1.5g
- Sodium: 50mg

Serves
- **4 servings**

Cooking Time
- **Total time: 20 minutes**

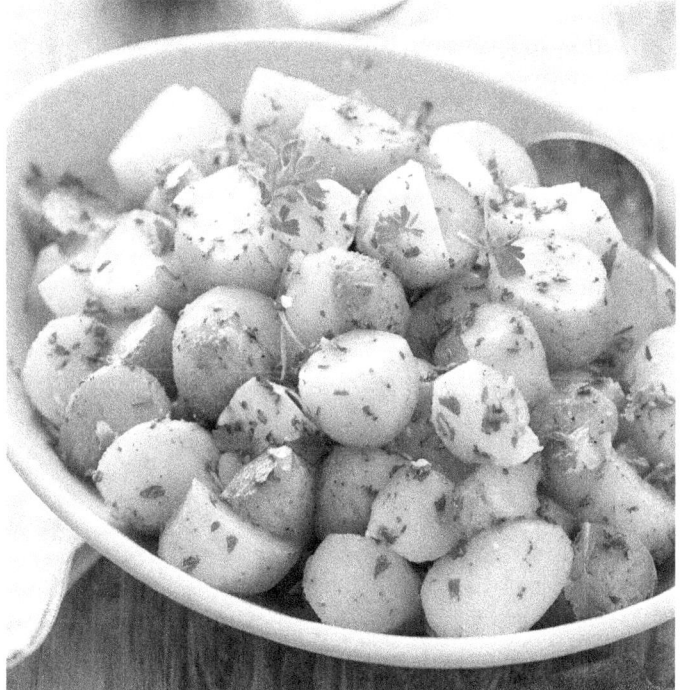

4. Spinach and Ricotta Stuffed Shells

Ingredients

- 12 jumbo pasta shells
- 2 cups fresh spinach, chopped
- 1 cup ricotta cheese
- 1/2 cup low-fat mozzarella cheese, shredded
- 1 tablespoon fresh basil, chopped
- 1 teaspoon dried oregano

Instructions

1. Preheat your oven to 350°F (175°C). Lightly grease a baking dish.
2. Cook the jumbo pasta shells according to package instructions. Drain and set aside.
3. In a large bowl, combine the chopped spinach, ricotta cheese, fresh basil, and dried oregano.
4. Stuff each pasta shell with the spinach and ricotta mixture and place them in the baking dish.
5. Sprinkle the shredded mozzarella cheese over the top.
6. Cover with foil and bake for 20 minutes.
7. Remove the foil and bake for an additional 10 minutes, or until the cheese is melted and bubbly.
8. Serve warm.

Nutrition Info (per serving)

- Calories: 220
- Protein: 12g
- Carbohydrates: 25g
- Fiber: 2g
- Sugars: 2g
- Fat: 9g
- Saturated Fat: 4g
- Sodium: 140mg

Serves

- **4 servings**

Cooking Time

- **Total time: 40 minutes**

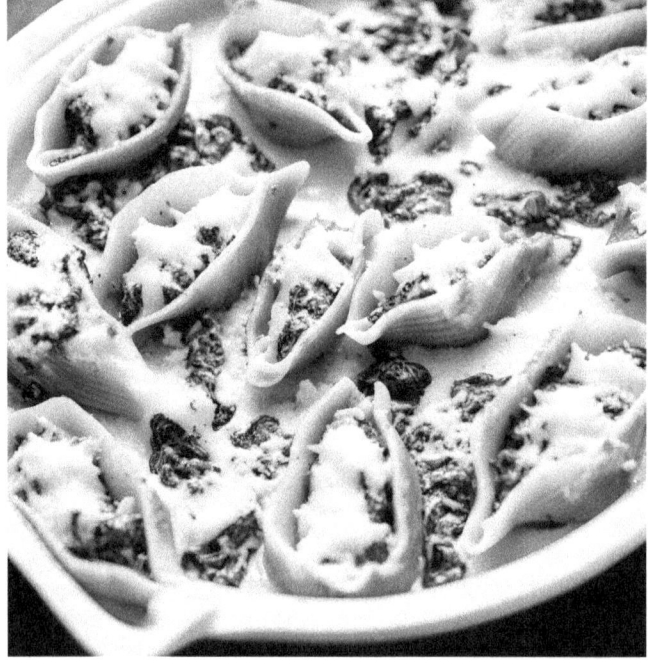

5. Mushroom and Barley Soup

Ingredients
- 1 cup barley
- 4 cups low-sodium vegetable broth
- 1 cup mushrooms, sliced
- 1 cup diced carrots
- 1 cup diced celery
- 2 tablespoons olive oil
- 1 teaspoon dried thyme
- 1 teaspoon dried parsley

Instructions
1. In a large pot, heat the olive oil over medium heat.
2. Add the diced carrots and celery, and cook for about 5 minutes until tender.
3. Add the mushrooms and cook for another 5 minutes.
4. Pour in the vegetable broth and bring to a boil.
5. Add the barley, dried thyme, and dried parsley.
6. Reduce the heat, cover, and simmer for 30-35 minutes, or until the barley is tender.
7. Serve warm.

Nutrition Info (per serving)
- Calories: 180
- Protein: 5g
- Carbohydrates: 30g
- Fiber: 5g
- Sugars: 5g
- Fat: 6g
- Saturated Fat: 1g
- Sodium: 180mg

Serves
- 4 servings

Cooking Time
- **Total time: 45 minutes**

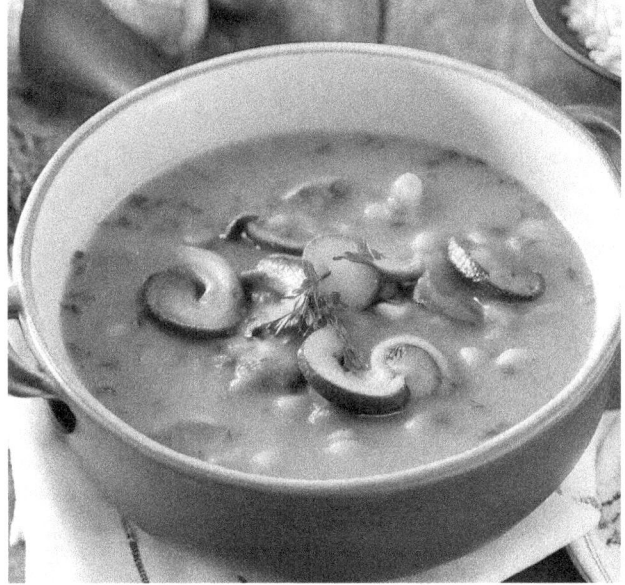

6. Oven-Roasted Kohlrabi

Ingredients
- 4 kohlrabi bulbs, peeled and cut into wedges
- 2 tablespoons olive oil
- 1 teaspoon dried thyme
- 1 teaspoon dried rosemary
- Fresh parsley, chopped (for garnish)

Instructions
1. Preheat your oven to 400°F (200°C). Line a baking sheet with parchment paper.
2. In a bowl, toss the kohlrabi wedges with olive oil, dried thyme, and dried rosemary.
3. Spread the kohlrabi wedges evenly on the prepared baking sheet.
4. Roast in the preheated oven for 25-30 minutes, or until the kohlrabi is tender and golden brown.
5. Remove from the oven and transfer to a serving plate.
6. Garnish with chopped fresh parsley and serve warm.

Nutrition Info (per serving)
- Calories: 120
- Protein: 2g
- Carbohydrates: 10g
- Fiber: 5g
- Sugars: 4g
- Fat: 8g
- Saturated Fat: 1g
- Sodium: 40mg

Serves
- 4 servings

Cooking Time
- **Total time: 30 minutes**

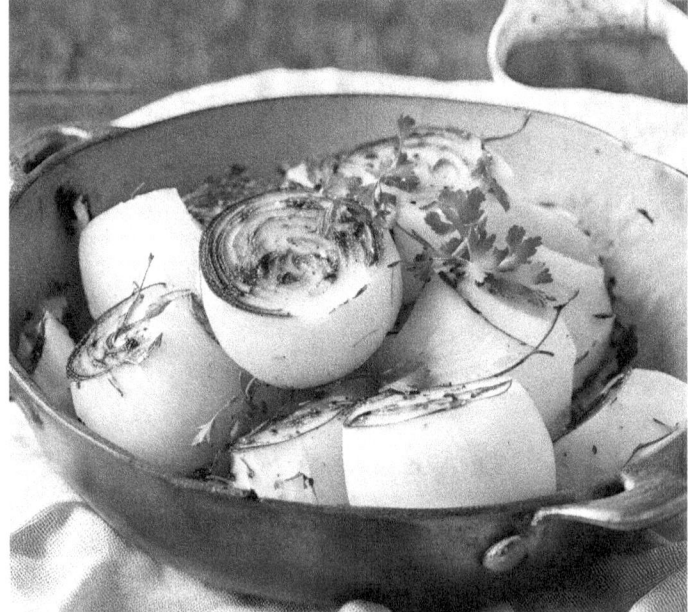

7. Cream of Mushroom Soup

Ingredients
- 2 cups mushrooms, sliced
- 2 cups low-sodium vegetable broth
- 1 cup low-fat milk
- 1 tablespoon olive oil
- 1 teaspoon dried thyme
- 1 teaspoon dried parsley
- 2 tablespoons all-purpose flour

Instructions
1. In a large pot, heat the olive oil over medium heat.
2. Add the sliced mushrooms and cook for about 5 minutes, until tender.
3. Sprinkle the flour over the mushrooms and stir to coat evenly.
4. Gradually add the vegetable broth, stirring constantly to avoid lumps.
5. Add the dried thyme and dried parsley.
6. Bring the mixture to a boil, then reduce the heat and simmer for 10 minutes.
7. Stir in the low-fat milk and cook for another 5 minutes, until the soup is heated through.
8. Serve warm.

Nutrition Info (per serving)
- Calories: 110
- Protein: 4g
- Carbohydrates: 12g
- Fiber: 2g
- Sugars: 4g
- Fat: 5g
- Saturated Fat: 1g
- Sodium: 80mg

Serves
- 4 servings

Cooking Time
- **Total time: 25 minutes**

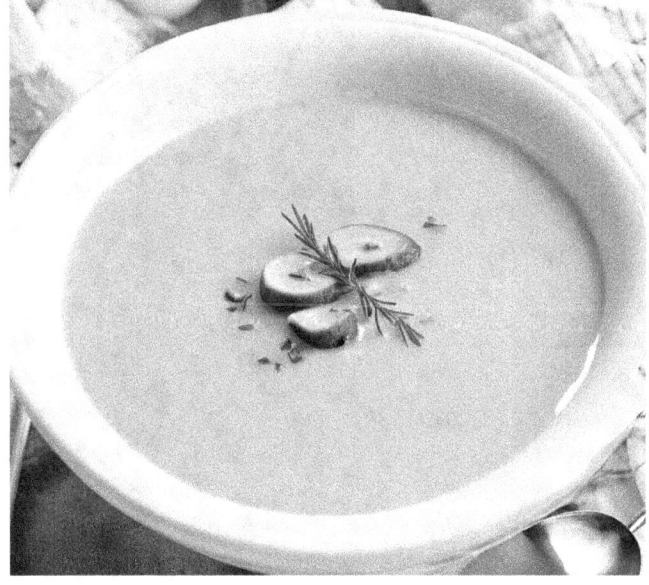

8. Vegetable Quinoa Pilaf

Ingredients
- 1 cup quinoa, rinsed
- 2 cups low-sodium vegetable broth
- 1 cup diced carrots
- 1 cup diced zucchini
- 1 cup peas
- 2 tablespoons olive oil
- 1 teaspoon dried basil
- 1 teaspoon dried oregano

Instructions
1. In a medium pot, bring the vegetable broth to a boil.
2. Add the rinsed quinoa, reduce the heat, cover, and simmer for 15 minutes, or until the quinoa is tender and the liquid is absorbed.
3. In a large skillet, heat the olive oil over medium heat.
4. Add the diced carrots and cook for 5 minutes, until they begin to soften.
5. Add the diced zucchini and peas, and cook for another 5 minutes, until all the vegetables are tender.
6. Stir in the cooked quinoa, dried basil, and dried oregano. Mix well to combine.
7. Serve warm.

Nutrition Info (per serving)
- Calories: 210
- Protein: 6g
- Carbohydrates: 30g
- Fiber: 5g
- Sugars: 4g
- Fat: 8g
- Saturated Fat: 1g
- Sodium: 90mg

Serves
- 4 servings

Cooking Time
- Total time: 25 minutes

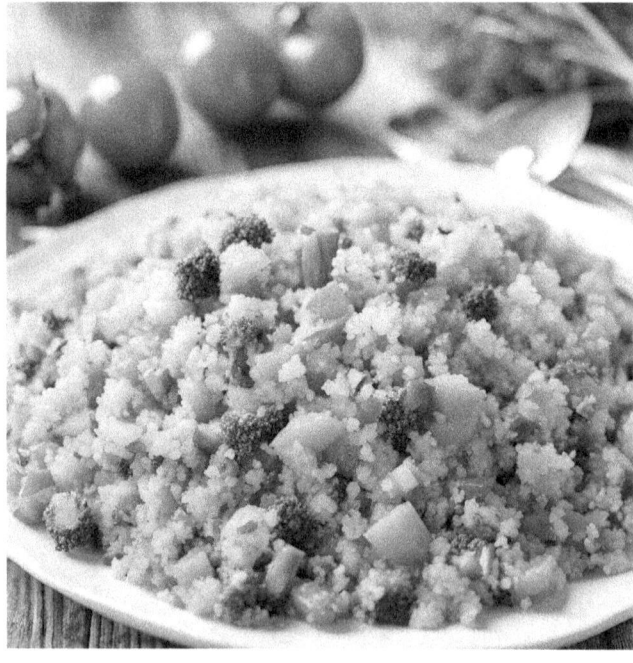

9. Fennel and Carrot Slaw

Ingredients
- 1 medium fennel bulb, thinly sliced
- 2 large carrots, peeled and shredded
- 2 tablespoons olive oil
- 1 tablespoon lemon juice (if tolerated)
- 1 teaspoon dried dill

Instructions
1. In a large bowl, combine the thinly sliced fennel and shredded carrots.
2. In a small bowl, whisk together the olive oil, lemon juice (if tolerated), and dried dill.
3. Pour the dressing over the fennel and carrots and toss to combine.
4. Serve immediately or refrigerate until ready to eat.

Nutrition Info (per serving)
- Calories: 80
- Protein: 1g
- Carbohydrates: 8g
- Fiber: 3g
- Sugars: 4g
- Fat: 5g
- Saturated Fat: 1g
- Sodium: 20mg

Serves
- **4 servings**

Cooking Time
- **Total time: 15 minutes**

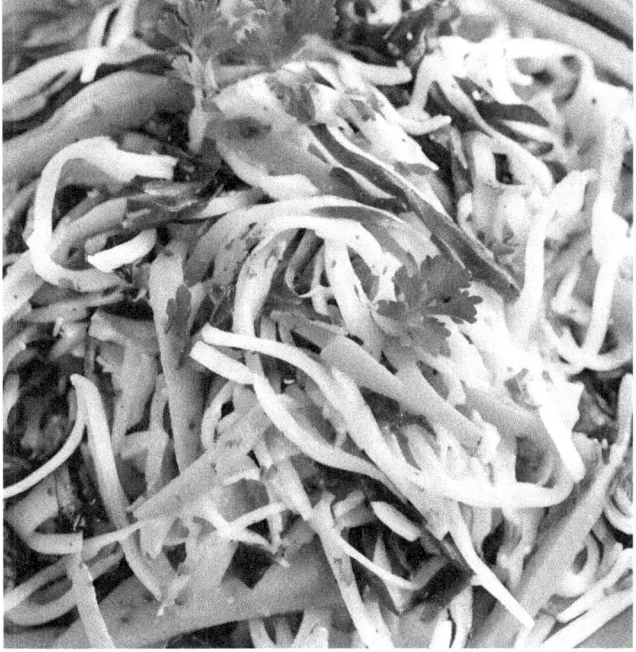

10. Sweet Pea and Potato Puree

Ingredients
- 2 large potatoes, peeled and diced
- 1 cup peas
- 1/2 cup low-fat milk or almond milk
- 1 tablespoon olive oil
- 1 teaspoon dried thyme

Instructions
1. In a large pot, bring the diced potatoes to a boil in salted water. Cook until tender, about 15 minutes.
2. Add the peas during the last 5 minutes of cooking.
3. Drain the potatoes and peas and return them to the pot.
4. Add the low-fat milk or almond milk, olive oil, and dried thyme.
5. Mash until smooth and creamy.
6. Serve warm.

Nutrition Info (per serving)
- Calories: 150
- Protein: 4g
- Carbohydrates: 28g
- Fiber: 4g
- Sugars: 5g
- Fat: 4g
- Saturated Fat: 1g
- Sodium: 30mg

Serves
- 4 servings

Cooking Time
- **Total time: 20 minutes**

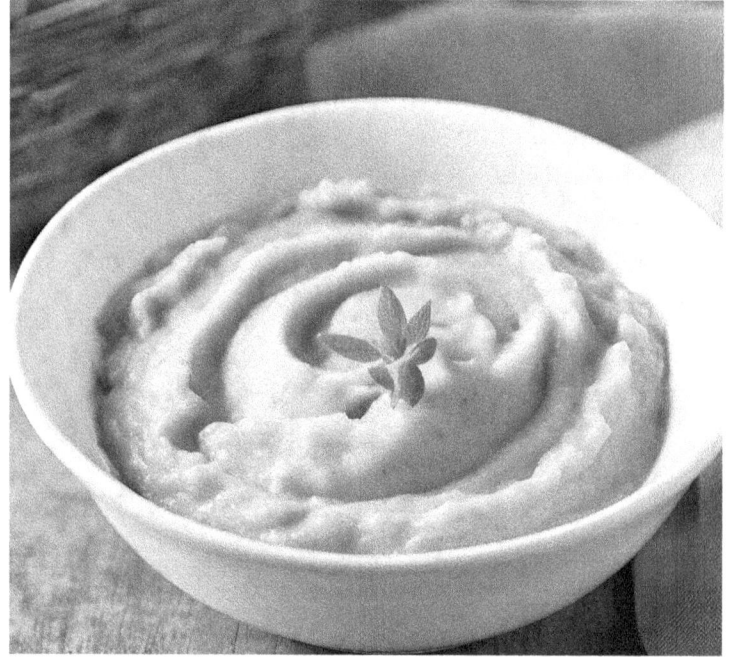

11. Green Bean Almondine

Ingredients
- 1 pound green beans, trimmed
- 2 tablespoons olive oil
- 1/4 cup sliced almonds
- 1 teaspoon dried basil
- 1 teaspoon dried oregano

Instructions
1. In a large pot, bring water to a boil. Add the green beans and cook for 4-5 minutes, until tender-crisp.
2. Drain the green beans and set aside.
3. In a large skillet, heat the olive oil over medium heat.
4. Add the sliced almonds and cook for 2-3 minutes, until lightly toasted.
5. Add the green beans, dried basil, and dried oregano to the skillet. Toss to combine and cook for an additional 2-3 minutes until heated through.
6. Serve warm.

Nutrition Info (per serving)
- Calories: 140
- Protein: 3g
- Carbohydrates: 8g
- Fiber: 4g
- Sugars: 3g
- Fat: 11g
- Saturated Fat: 1.5g
- Sodium: 20mg

Serves
- 4 servings

Cooking Time
- **Total time: 15 minutes**

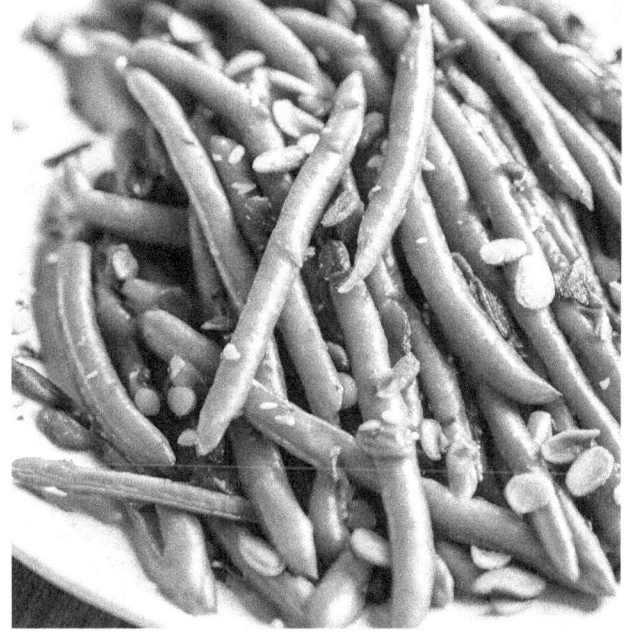

12. Stuffed Zucchini

Ingredients
- 4 medium zucchinis, halved lengthwise and seeds scooped out
- 1 cup cooked quinoa
- 1/2 cup diced tomatoes (if tolerated)
- 1/4 cup low-fat mozzarella cheese, shredded
- 1 tablespoon olive oil
- 1 teaspoon dried basil
- 1 teaspoon dried oregano

Instructions
1. Preheat your oven to 375°F (190°C). Lightly grease a baking dish.
2. In a bowl, mix together the cooked quinoa, diced tomatoes (if tolerated), shredded mozzarella cheese, olive oil, dried basil, and dried oregano.
3. Fill each zucchini half with the quinoa mixture and place them in the baking dish.
4. Cover with foil and bake for 20 minutes.
5. Remove the foil and bake for an additional 10 minutes, or until the zucchinis are tender and the cheese is melted and golden brown.
6. Serve warm.

Nutrition Info (per serving)
- Calories: 180
- Protein: 8g
- Carbohydrates: 20g
- Fiber: 4g
- Sugars: 4g
- Fat: 8g
- Saturated Fat: 2g
- Sodium: 60mg

Serves
- **4 servings**

Cooking Time
- **Total time: 30 minutes**

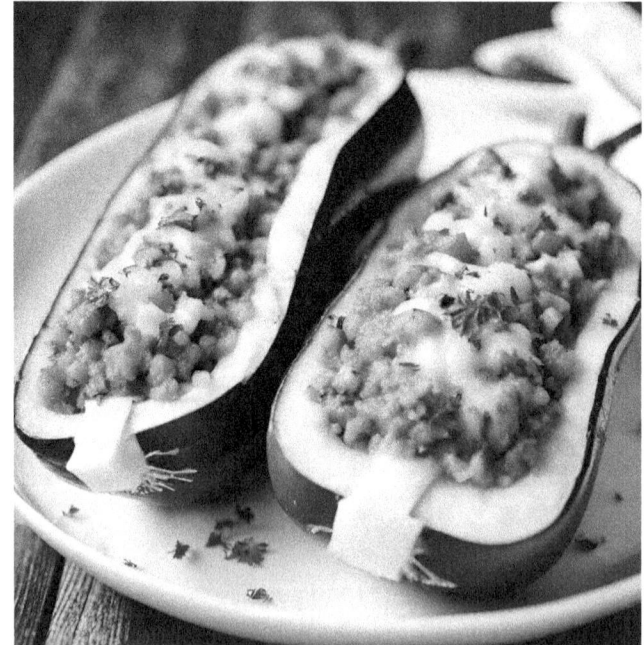

13. Leek and Potato Soup

Ingredients
- 2 large leeks, white and light green parts only, sliced
- 4 medium potatoes, peeled and diced
- 4 cups low-sodium vegetable broth
- 1 cup low-fat milk or almond milk
- 2 tablespoons olive oil
- 1 teaspoon dried thyme

Instructions
1. In a large pot, heat the olive oil over medium heat.
2. Add the sliced leeks and cook for about 5 minutes, until they are softened.
3. Add the diced potatoes and cook for another 5 minutes, stirring occasionally.
4. Pour in the vegetable broth and bring to a boil.
5. Reduce the heat, cover, and simmer for 20 minutes, or until the potatoes are tender.
6. Use an immersion blender to puree the soup until smooth, or transfer to a blender in batches.
7. Stir in the low-fat milk or almond milk and dried thyme.
8. Cook for another 5 minutes until heated through.
9. Serve warm.

Nutrition Info (per serving)
- Calories: 150
- Protein: 4g
- Carbohydrates: 28g
- Fiber: 4g
- Sugars: 3g
- Fat: 4g
- Saturated Fat: 1g
- Sodium: 100mg

Serves
- **4 servings**

Cooking Time
- **Total time: 35 minutes**

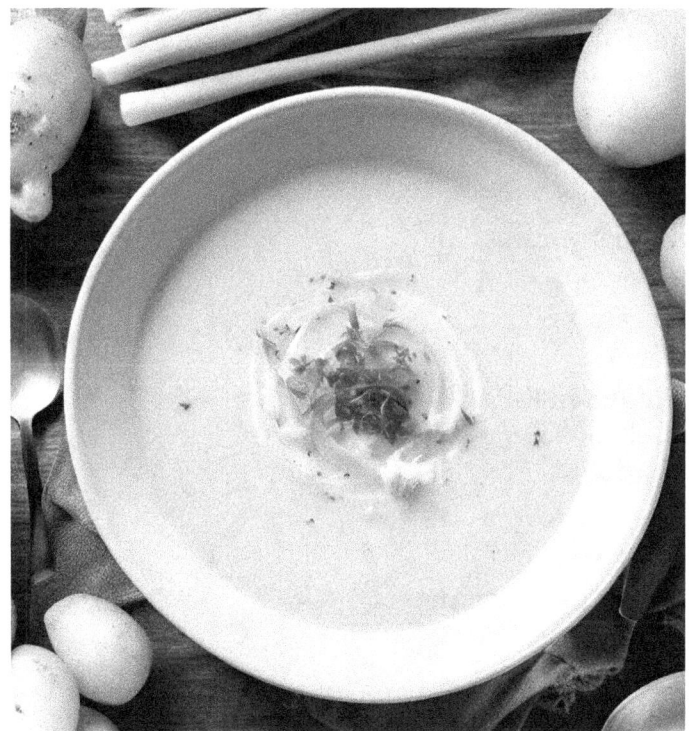

14. Butternut Squash Risotto

Ingredients
- 1 cup Arborio rice
- 2 cups diced butternut squash
- 4 cups low-sodium vegetable broth
- 1 cup low-fat milk
- 2 tablespoons olive oil
- 1 teaspoon dried sage
- 1 teaspoon dried thyme

Instructions
1. In a medium pot, heat the vegetable broth over low heat to keep it warm.
2. In a large pot, heat the olive oil over medium heat.
3. Add the diced butternut squash and cook for about 5 minutes, until it begins to soften.
4. Add the Arborio rice and cook for another 2 minutes, stirring constantly to coat the rice with the oil.
5. Begin adding the warm vegetable broth, one ladle at a time, stirring frequently. Wait until most of the broth is absorbed before adding the next ladle.
6. Continue this process until the rice is creamy and cooked through, about 18-20 minutes.
7. Stir in the low-fat milk, dried sage, and dried thyme. Cook for another 5 minutes until heated through.
8. Serve warm.

Nutrition Info (per serving)
- Calories: 220
- Protein: 5g
- Carbohydrates: 40g
- Fiber: 3g
- Sugars: 4g
- Fat: 5g
- Saturated Fat: 1g
- Sodium: 140mg

Serves
- **4 servings**

Cooking Time
- **Total time: 30 minutes**

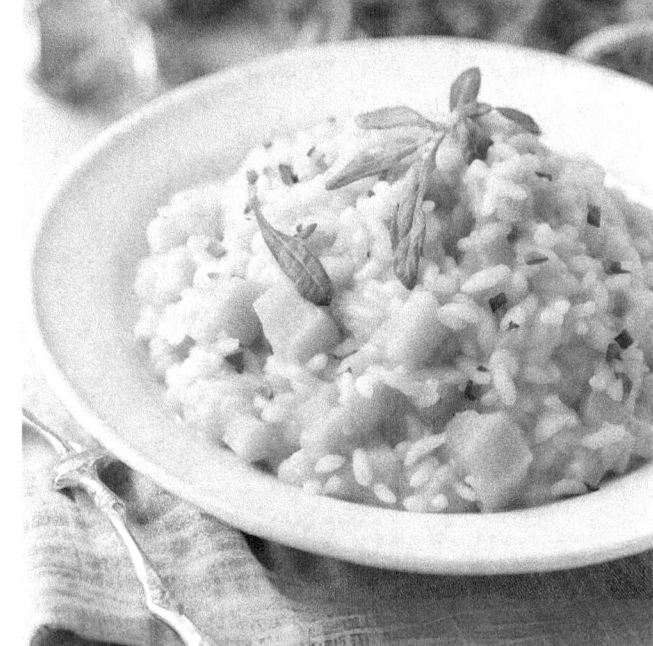

15. Roasted Parsnips

Ingredients
- 4 medium parsnips, peeled and cut into sticks
- 2 tablespoons olive oil
- 1 teaspoon dried thyme
- 1 teaspoon dried rosemary

Instructions
1. Preheat your oven to 400°F (200°C). Line a baking sheet with parchment paper.
2. In a bowl, toss the parsnip sticks with olive oil, dried thyme, and dried rosemary.
3. Spread the parsnips evenly on the prepared baking sheet.
4. Roast in the preheated oven for 25-30 minutes, or until the parsnips are tender and golden brown.
5. Serve warm.

Nutrition Info (per serving)
- Calories: 110
- Protein: 1g
- Carbohydrates: 15g
- Fiber: 5g
- Sugars: 5g
- Fat: 6g
- Saturated Fat: 1g
- Sodium: 20mg

Serves
- 4 servings

Cooking Time
- **Total time: 30 minutes**

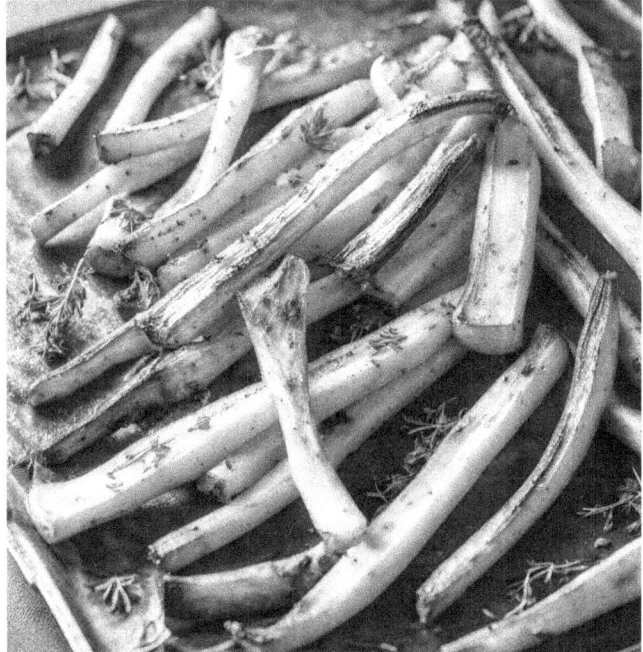

16. Carrot and Coriander Soup

Ingredients
- 6 large carrots, peeled and chopped
- 1 large leek, white and light green parts only, sliced
- 4 cups low-sodium vegetable broth
- 1 tablespoon olive oil
- 1 teaspoon ground coriander
- Fresh coriander, chopped (for garnish)

Instructions
1. In a large pot, heat the olive oil over medium heat.
2. Add the sliced leek and cook for about 5 minutes, until softened.
3. Add the chopped carrots and cook for another 5 minutes.
4. Pour in the vegetable broth and bring to a boil.
5. Reduce the heat, cover, and simmer for 20 minutes, or until the carrots are tender.
6. Use an immersion blender to puree the soup until smooth, or transfer to a blender in batches.
7. Stir in the ground coriander and cook for another 5 minutes until heated through.
8. Serve warm, garnished with chopped fresh coriander.

Nutrition Info (per serving)
- Calories: 100
- Protein: 2g
- Carbohydrates: 20g
- Fiber: 5g
- Sugars: 10g
- Fat: 3g
- Saturated Fat: 0.5g
- Sodium: 80mg

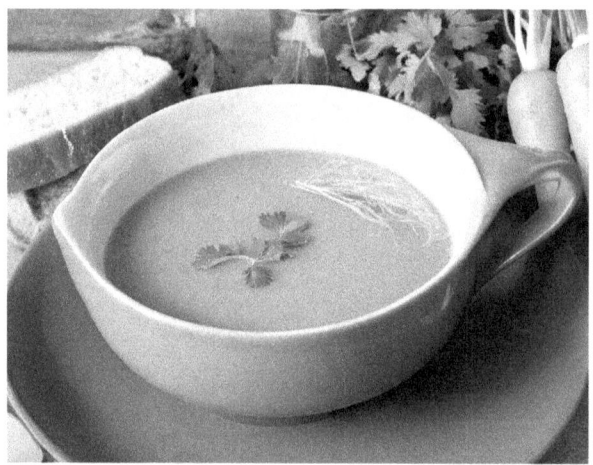

Serves
- 4 servings

Cooking Time
- **Total time: 35 minutes**

17. Celery Root Mash

Ingredients
- 2 large celery roots (celeriac), peeled and diced
- 2 medium potatoes, peeled and diced
- 1/2 cup low-fat milk or almond milk
- 2 tablespoons olive oil
- 1 teaspoon dried thyme

Instructions
1. In a large pot, bring the diced celery root and potatoes to a boil in salted water. Cook until tender, about 15-20 minutes.
2. Drain and return to the pot.
3. Add the low-fat milk or almond milk, olive oil, and dried thyme.
4. Mash until smooth and creamy.
5. Serve warm.

Nutrition Info (per serving)
- Calories: 130
- Protein: 2g
- Carbohydrates: 20g
- Fiber: 3g
- Sugars: 3g
- Fat: 5g
- Saturated Fat: 1g
- Sodium: 40mg

Serves
- 4 servings

Cooking Time
- **Total time: 25 minutes**

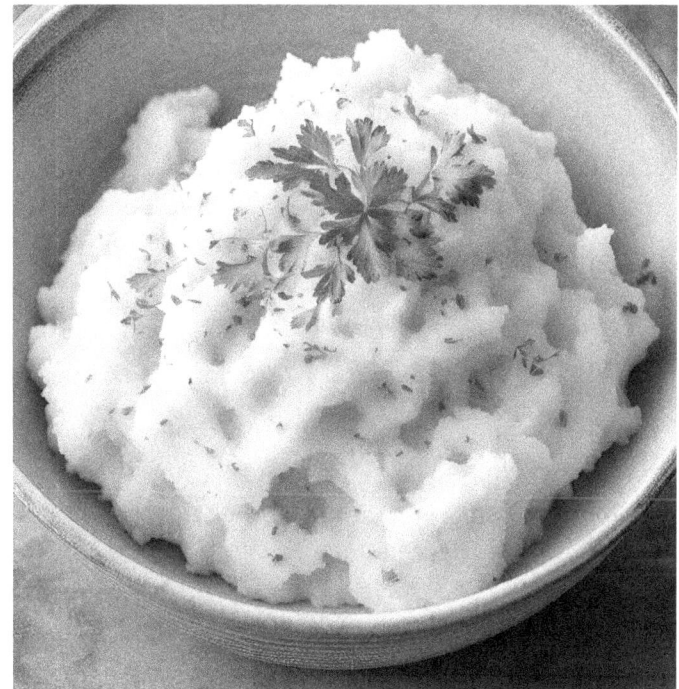

18. Steamed Brussels Sprouts

Ingredients
- 1 pound Brussels sprouts, trimmed and halved
- 2 tablespoons olive oil
- 1 teaspoon dried basil
- 1 teaspoon dried oregano

Instructions
1. In a large pot, bring 1-2 inches of water to a boil.
2. Place the Brussels sprouts in a steamer basket and set over the boiling water.
3. Cover and steam for 8-10 minutes, until tender.
4. Transfer the steamed Brussels sprouts to a bowl.
5. Drizzle with olive oil and sprinkle with dried basil and dried oregano. Toss to coat.
6. Serve warm.

Nutrition Info (per serving)
- Calories: 90
- Protein: 3g
- Carbohydrates: 9g
- Fiber: 4g
- Sugars: 2g
- Fat: 6g
- Saturated Fat: 1g
- Sodium: 20mg

Serves
- 4 servings

Cooking Time
- **Total time: 15 minutes**

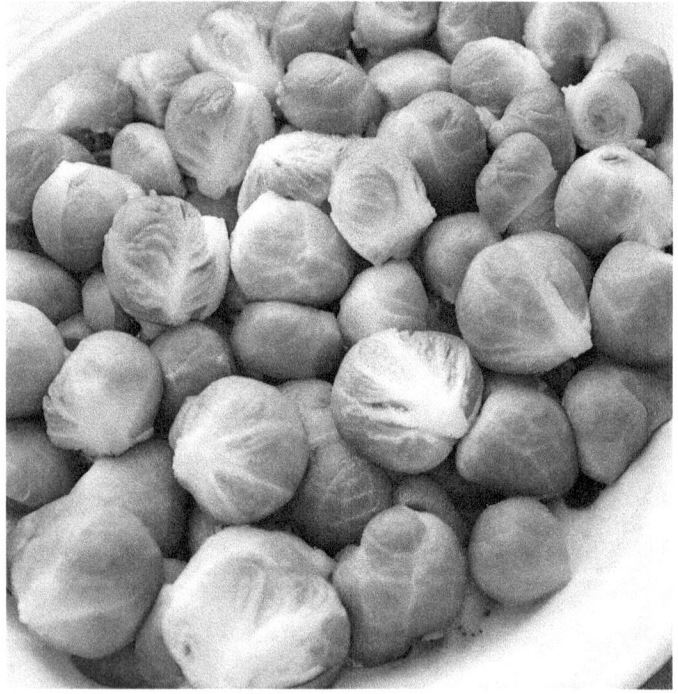

19. Stewed Green Beans

Ingredients
- 1 pound green beans, trimmed
- 1 cup diced carrots
- 2 cups low-sodium vegetable broth
- 2 tablespoons olive oil
- 1 teaspoon dried thyme
- 1 teaspoon dried rosemary

Instructions
1. In a large pot, heat the olive oil over medium heat.
2. Add the diced carrots and cook for about 5 minutes, until they begin to soften.
3. Add the green beans, vegetable broth, dried thyme, and dried rosemary.
4. Bring to a boil, then reduce the heat, cover, and simmer for 20-25 minutes, or until the green beans are tender.
5. Serve warm.

Nutrition Info (per serving)
- Calories: 100
- Protein: 2g
- Carbohydrates: 10g
- Fiber: 4g
- Sugars: 4g
- Fat: 6g
- Saturated Fat: 1g
- Sodium: 140mg

Serves
- **4 servings**

Cooking Time
- **Total time: 30 minutes**

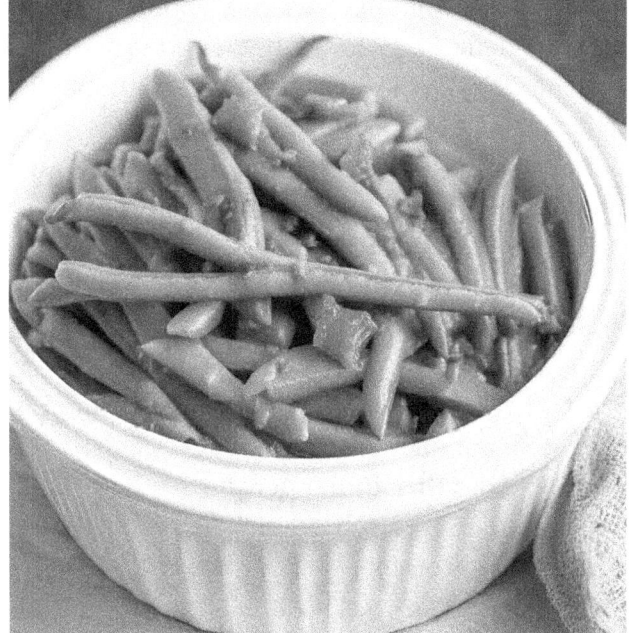

Desserts

1. Carrot Cake

Ingredients
- 2 cups grated carrots
- 1 1/2 cups whole wheat flour
- 1 teaspoon baking powder
- 1/2 teaspoon baking soda
- 1 teaspoon ground cinnamon
- 1/2 teaspoon ground ginger
- 1/4 teaspoon ground nutmeg
- 3/4 cup applesauce
- 1/2 cup honey
- 2 large eggs
- 1/2 cup low-fat Greek yogurt
- 1 teaspoon vanilla extract

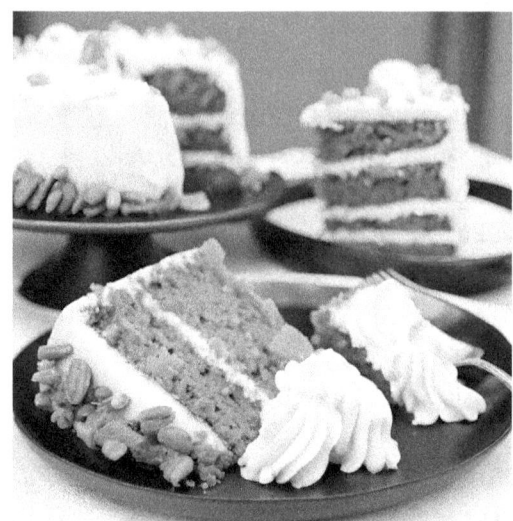

Instructions
1. Preheat your oven to 350°F (175°C). Grease and flour a 9-inch round cake pan.
2. In a large bowl, mix together the whole wheat flour, baking powder, baking soda, ground cinnamon, ground ginger, and ground nutmeg.
3. In another bowl, whisk together the applesauce, honey, eggs, Greek yogurt, and vanilla extract until well combined.
4. Gradually add the wet ingredients to the dry ingredients, mixing until just combined.
5. Fold in the grated carrots.
6. Pour the batter into the prepared cake pan and spread evenly.
7. Bake for 30-35 minutes, or until a toothpick inserted into the center comes out clean.
8. Allow the cake to cool in the pan for 10 minutes before transferring to a wire rack to cool completely.
9. Serve warm or at room temperature.

Nutrition Info (per serving)
- Calories: 180   Protein: 5g   Carbohydrates: 32g   Fiber: 3g
- Sugars: 18g   Fat: 4g   Saturated Fat: 1g
- Sodium: 160mg

Serves
- 8 servings

Cooking Time
- Total time: 45 minutes

2. Mango Mousse

Ingredients
- 2 large ripe mangoes, peeled and diced
- 1 cup low-fat Greek yogurt
- 1 tablespoon honey
- 1 teaspoon vanilla extract
- 1 tablespoon unflavored gelatin
- 1/4 cup water

Instructions
1. In a blender or food processor, puree the diced mangoes until smooth.
2. In a small bowl, sprinkle the gelatin over the water and let it sit for a few minutes to soften.
3. Heat the gelatin mixture in the microwave for about 10 seconds, or until fully dissolved.
4. In a large bowl, whisk together the Greek yogurt, honey, and vanilla extract.
5. Stir in the mango puree and dissolved gelatin until well combined.
6. Pour the mixture into serving dishes and refrigerate for at least 2 hours, or until set.
7. Serve chilled.

Nutrition Info (per serving)
- Calories: 120
- Protein: 5g
- Carbohydrates: 25g
- Fiber: 2g
- Sugars: 22g
- Fat: 1g
- Saturated Fat: 0.5g
- Sodium: 30mg

Serves
- 4 servings

Cooking Time
- **Total time: 2 hours 15 minutes (including chilling time)**

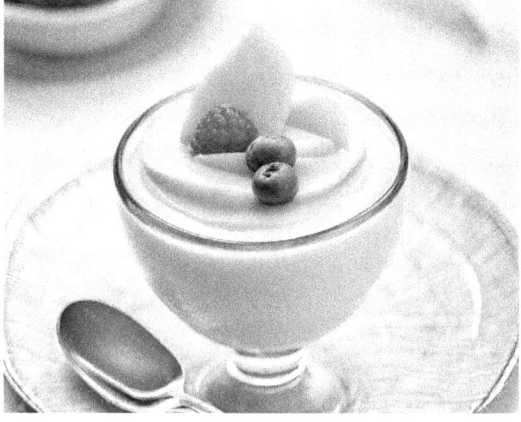

3. Vanilla and Honey Panna Cotta

Ingredients
- 2 cups low-fat milk
- 1/4 cup honey
- 2 teaspoons vanilla extract
- 2 tablespoons unflavored gelatin
- 1/4 cup water

Instructions
1. In a small bowl, sprinkle the gelatin over the water and let it sit for a few minutes to soften.
2. In a medium saucepan, combine the milk and honey. Heat over medium heat until the mixture is hot but not boiling.
3. Remove from heat and stir in the softened gelatin until fully dissolved.
4. Stir in the vanilla extract.
5. Pour the mixture into ramekins or serving dishes.
6. Refrigerate for at least 4 hours, or until set.
7. Serve chilled.

Nutrition Info (per serving)
- Calories: 110
- Protein: 6g
- Carbohydrates: 20g
- Fiber: 0g
- Sugars: 18g
- Fat: 1g
- Saturated Fat: 0.5g
- Sodium: 40mg

Serves
- 4 servings

Cooking Time
- **Total time: 4 hours 15 minutes (including chilling time)**

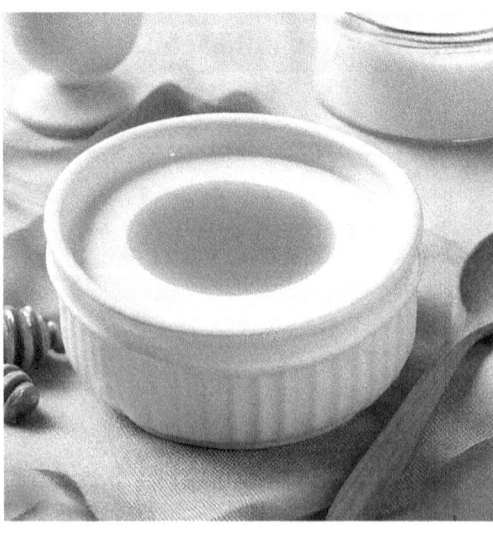

4. Banana Ice Cream

Ingredients
- 4 ripe bananas, peeled and sliced
- 1/4 cup low-fat Greek yogurt
- 1 tablespoon honey
- 1 teaspoon vanilla extract

Instructions
1. Place the sliced bananas in a single layer on a baking sheet and freeze for at least 2 hours, or until completely frozen.
2. In a blender or food processor, combine the frozen bananas, Greek yogurt, honey, and vanilla extract.
3. Blend until smooth and creamy, scraping down the sides as needed.
4. Serve immediately for a soft-serve consistency or transfer to a container and freeze for an additional 1-2 hours for a firmer texture.
5. Serve chilled.

Nutrition Info (per serving)
- Calories: 100
- Protein: 2g
- Carbohydrates: 25g
- Fiber: 3g
- Sugars: 18g
- Fat: 0.5g
- Saturated Fat: 0g
- Sodium: 5mg

Serves
- **4 servings**

Cooking Time
- **Total time: 2 hours 10 minutes (including freezing time)**

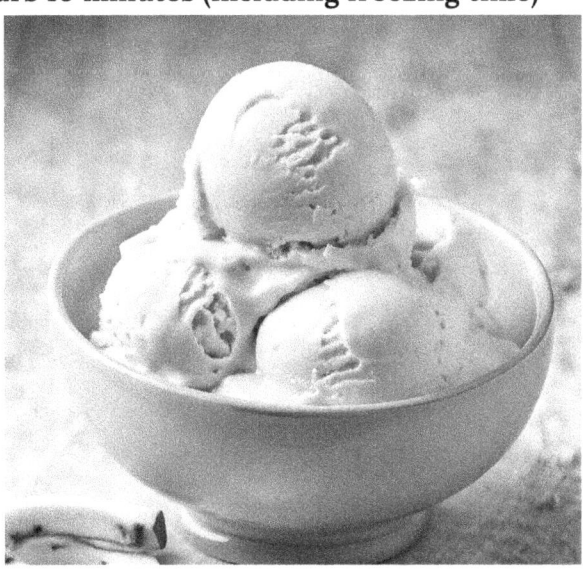

5. Warm Apple Cider

Ingredients
- 4 cups apple cider
- 1 cinnamon stick
- 1 teaspoon ground ginger
- 1 teaspoon ground nutmeg
- 1 tablespoon honey

Instructions
1. In a large saucepan, combine the apple cider, cinnamon stick, ground ginger, and ground nutmeg.
2. Heat over medium heat until the mixture is hot but not boiling.
3. Stir in the honey until dissolved.
4. Remove from heat and let the cider sit for a few minutes to allow the flavors to blend.
5. Remove the cinnamon stick and pour the cider into mugs.
6. Serve warm.

Nutrition Info (per serving)
- Calories: 100
- Protein: 0g
- Carbohydrates: 25g
- Fiber: 0g
- Sugars: 24g
- Fat: 0g
- Saturated Fat: 0g
- Sodium: 5mg

Serves
- 4 servings

Cooking Time
- **Total time: 15 minutes**

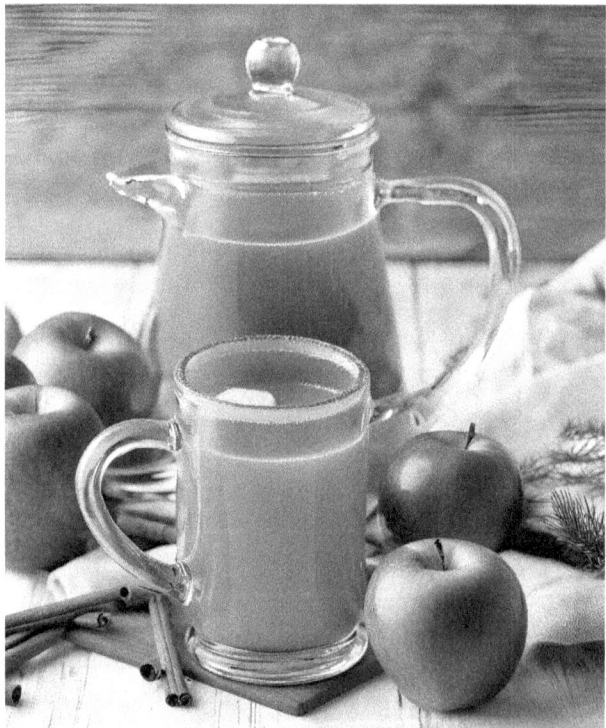

6. Oatmeal Smoothie

Ingredients

- 1/2 cup rolled oats
- 1 cup low-fat milk or almond milk
- 1 ripe banana
- 1 tablespoon honey
- 1 teaspoon vanilla extract

Instructions

1. In a blender, combine the rolled oats, milk, banana, honey, and vanilla extract.
2. Blend until smooth and creamy.
3. Pour into glasses and serve immediately.

Nutrition Info (per serving)

- Calories: 180
- Protein: 5g
- Carbohydrates: 35g
- Fiber: 4g
- Sugars: 18g
- Fat: 3g
- Saturated Fat: 0.5g
- Sodium: 40mg

Serves

- 2 servings

Cooking Time

- **Total time: 5 minutes**

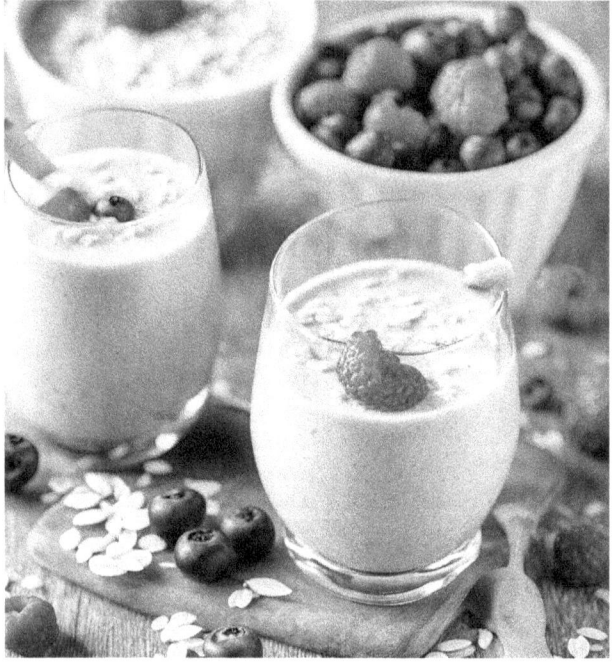

10-WEEK MEAL PLAN

Week 1
Monday
- Breakfast: Oatmeal Porridge
- Lunch: Chicken and Avocado Salad
- Dinner: Steamed Cod with Zucchini
- Snack: Carrot Juice

Tuesday
- Breakfast: Banana Yogurt Smoothie
- Lunch: Vegetable Stew
- Dinner: Poached Salmon with Steamed Brussels Sprouts
- Snack: Warm Apple Cider

Wednesday
- Breakfast: Boiled Sweet Potatoes
- Lunch: Turkey and Sweet Potato Hash
- Dinner: Baked Tilapia with Minted Peas
- Snack: Pear and Yogurt Smoothie

Thursday
- Breakfast: Cottage Cheese with Melon
- Lunch: Spinach and Ricotta Stuffed Shells
- Dinner: Grilled Shrimp with Green Beans Almondine
- Snack: Oatmeal Smoothie

Friday
- Breakfast: Mashed Potatoes
- Lunch: Stewed Green Beans
- Dinner: Baked Sea Bass with Roasted Parsnips
- Snack: Peach Smoothie

Saturday
- Breakfast: Pumpkin Porridge
- Lunch: Herbed Potato Salad
- Dinner: Chicken and Parsnip Stew
- Snack: Mango Mousse

Sunday
- Breakfast: Vegetable Omelet
- Lunch: Stuffed Zucchini
- Dinner: Salmon and Potato Bake
- Snack: Banana Ice Cream

Week 2

Monday
- Breakfast: Smoothie Bowl
- Lunch: Clam and Potato Casserole
- Dinner: Oven-Poached Flounder with Carrot and Coriander Soup
- Snack: Vanilla and Honey Panna Cotta

Tuesday
- Breakfast: Polenta
- Lunch: Turkey Vegetable Loaf
- Dinner: Scallops with Parsnip Puree
- Snack: Carrot Cake

Wednesday
- Breakfast: Carrot and Ginger Juice
- Lunch: Sweet Pea and Potato Puree
- Dinner: Halibut and Zucchini
- Snack: Warm Apple Cider

Thursday
- Breakfast: Squash Soup
- Lunch: Baked Chicken and Mushrooms
- Dinner: Shrimp and Rice Pilaf
- Snack: Mango Mousse

Friday
- Breakfast: Steamed Vegetables
- Lunch: Turkey and Oat Porridge
- Dinner: Poached Pear and Salmon
- Snack: Pear and Yogurt Smoothie

Saturday
- Breakfast: Quinoa Salad
- Lunch: Herbed Turkey Steaks
- Dinner: Clam Soup
- Snack: Carrot Juice

Sunday
- Breakfast: Sweet Potato Hash
- Lunch: Spinach and Ricotta Stuffed Shells
- Dinner: Grilled Sole with Green Bean Almondine
- Snack: Banana Ice Cream

Week 3

Monday
- Breakfast: Almond Rice Porridge
- Lunch: Chicken and Peas Pilaf
- Dinner: Baked Haddock with Stewed Green Beans
- Snack: Peach Smoothie

Tuesday
- Breakfast: Soft Boiled Eggs
- Lunch: Vegetable Quinoa Pilaf
- Dinner: Scallop Soup
- Snack: Oatmeal Smoothie

Wednesday
- Breakfast: Barley Soup
- Lunch: Baked Turkey and Eggplant
- Dinner: Tilapia with Minted Peas
- Snack: Vanilla and Honey Panna Cotta

Thursday
- Breakfast: Omelet with Herbs
- Lunch: Steamed Brussels Sprouts
- Dinner: Ginger Shrimp Stir Fry
- Snack: Mango Mousse

Friday
- Breakfast: Zucchini Bread
- Lunch: Herbed Potato Salad
- Dinner: Turkey and Squash Skillet
- Snack: Pear and Yogurt Smoothie

Saturday
- Breakfast: Millet Porridge
- Lunch: Chicken Porridge
- Dinner: Cod and Asparagus Bake
- Snack: Carrot Cake

Sunday
- Breakfast: Pear Smoothie
- Lunch: Carrot and Coriander Soup
- Dinner: Grilled Shrimp with Green Beans Almondine
- Snack: Warm Apple Cider

Week 4

Monday
- Breakfast: Buckwheat Pancakes
- Lunch: Stewed Green Beans
- Dinner: Poached Salmon with Steamed Brussels Sprouts
- Snack: Banana Ice Cream

Tuesday
- Breakfast: Rye Bread Sandwich
- Lunch: Chicken and Avocado Salad
- Dinner: Baked Sea Bass with Roasted Parsnips
- Snack: Oatmeal Smoothie

Wednesday
- Breakfast: Basil and Spinach Smoothie
- Lunch: Spinach and Ricotta Stuffed Shells
- Dinner: Clam and Potato Casserole
- Snack: Pear and Yogurt Smoothie

Thursday
- Breakfast: Turkey and Sweet Potato Hash
- Lunch: Stuffed Zucchini
- Dinner: Halibut and Zucchini
- Snack: Peach Smoothie

Friday
- Breakfast: Oatmeal Smoothie
- Lunch: Herbed Turkey Steaks
- Dinner: Shrimp and Rice Pilaf
- Snack: Warm Apple Cider

Saturday
- Breakfast: Carrot Juice
- Lunch: Sweet Pea and Potato Puree
- Dinner: Scallops with Parsnip Puree
- Snack: Mango Mousse

Sunday
- Breakfast: Smoothie Bowl
- Lunch: Vegetable Quinoa Pilaf
- Dinner: Oven-Poached Flounder with Carrot and Coriander Soup
- Snack: Vanilla and Honey Panna Cotta

Week 5

Monday
- Breakfast: Quinoa Salad
- Lunch: Chicken and Parsnip Stew
- Dinner: Baked Haddock with Stewed Green Beans
- Snack: Carrot Cake

Tuesday
- Breakfast: Sweet Potato Hash
- Lunch: Herbed Potato Salad
- Dinner: Tilapia with Minted Peas
- Snack: Banana Ice Cream

Wednesday
- Breakfast: Almond Rice Porridge
- Lunch: Steamed Brussels Sprouts
- Dinner: Ginger Shrimp Stir Fry
- Snack: Pear and Yogurt Smoothie

Thursday
- Breakfast: Soft Boiled Eggs
- Lunch: Baked Turkey and Eggplant
- Dinner: Turkey and Squash Skillet
- Snack: Peach Smoothie

Friday
- Breakfast: Barley Soup
- Lunch: Chicken Porridge
- Dinner: Cod and Asparagus Bake
- Snack: Oatmeal Smoothie

Saturday
- Breakfast: Omelet with Herbs
- Lunch: Carrot and Coriander Soup
- Dinner: Grilled Shrimp with Green Beans Almondine
- Snack: Mango Mousse

Sunday
- Breakfast: Zucchini Bread
- Lunch: Spinach and Ricotta Stuffed Shells
- Dinner: Scallop Soup
- Snack: Vanilla and Honey Panna Cotta

Week 6

Monday
- Breakfast: Pumpkin Porridge
- Lunch: Turkey and Oat Porridge
- Dinner: Steamed Cod with Stewed Green Beans
- Snack: Vanilla and Honey Panna Cotta

Tuesday
- Breakfast: Banana Yogurt Smoothie
- Lunch: Herbed Potato Salad
- Dinner: Baked Tilapia with Minted Peas
- Snack: Carrot Cake

Wednesday
- Breakfast: Boiled Sweet Potatoes
- Lunch: Vegetable Quinoa Pilaf
- Dinner: Poached Salmon with Steamed Brussels Sprouts
- Snack: Mango Mousse

Thursday
- Breakfast: Cottage Cheese with Melon
- Lunch: Sweet Pea and Potato Puree
- Dinner: Ginger Shrimp Stir Fry
- Snack: Oatmeal Smoothie

Friday
- Breakfast: Mashed Potatoes
- Lunch: Steamed Brussels Sprouts
- Dinner: Cod and Asparagus Bake
- Snack: Pear and Yogurt Smoothie

Saturday
- Breakfast: Carrot and Ginger Juice
- Lunch: Turkey and Sweet Potato Hash
- Dinner: Halibut and Zucchini
- Snack: Warm Apple Cider

Sunday
- Breakfast: Omelet with Herbs
- Lunch: Spinach and Ricotta Stuffed Shells
- Dinner: Clam and Potato Casserole
- Snack: Banana Ice Cream

Week 7

Monday
- Breakfast: Quinoa Salad
- Lunch: Chicken Porridge
- Dinner: Baked Sea Bass with Roasted Parsnips
- Snack: Peach Smoothie

Tuesday
- Breakfast: Soft Boiled Eggs
- Lunch: Stuffed Zucchini
- Dinner: Shrimp and Rice Pilaf
- Snack: Carrot Juice

Wednesday
- Breakfast: Barley Soup
- Lunch: Herbed Turkey Steaks
- Dinner: Scallops with Parsnip Puree
- Snack: Mango Mousse

Thursday
- Breakfast: Rye Bread Sandwich
- Lunch: Carrot and Coriander Soup
- Dinner: Tilapia with Minted Peas
- Snack: Vanilla and Honey Panna Cotta

Friday
- Breakfast: Basil and Spinach Smoothie
- Lunch: Chicken and Avocado Salad
- Dinner: Oven-Poached Flounder with Stewed Green Beans
- Snack: Banana Ice Cream

Saturday
- Breakfast: Turkey and Sweet Potato Hash
- Lunch: Vegetable Quinoa Pilaf
- Dinner: Grilled Shrimp with Green Beans Almondine
- Snack: Oatmeal Smoothie

Sunday
- Breakfast: Oatmeal Smoothie
- Lunch: Stewed Green Beans
- Dinner: Poached Salmon with Steamed Brussels Sprouts
- Snack: Pear and Yogurt Smoothie

Week 8

Monday
- Breakfast: Smoothie Bowl
- Lunch: Herbed Potato Salad
- Dinner: Scallop Soup
- Snack: Carrot Cake

Tuesday
- Breakfast: Millet Porridge
- Lunch: Turkey and Oat Porridge
- Dinner: Poached Pear and Salmon
- Snack: Warm Apple Cider

Wednesday
- Breakfast: Pear Smoothie
- Lunch: Stuffed Zucchini
- Dinner: Clam Soup
- Snack: Mango Mousse

Thursday
- Breakfast: Buckwheat Pancakes
- Lunch: Turkey and Sweet Potato Hash
- Dinner: Halibut and Zucchini
- Snack: Peach Smoothie

Friday
- Breakfast: Zucchini Bread
- Lunch: Chicken and Parsnip Stew
- Dinner: Baked Haddock with Stewed Green Beans
- Snack: Pear and Yogurt Smoothie

Saturday
- Breakfast: Carrot Juice
- Lunch: Steamed Brussels Sprouts
- Dinner: Ginger Shrimp Stir Fry
- Snack: Vanilla and Honey Panna Cotta

Sunday
- Breakfast: Omelet with Herbs
- Lunch: Spinach and Ricotta Stuffed Shells
- Dinner: Baked Sea Bass with Roasted Parsnips
- Snack: Banana Ice Cream

Week 9

Monday
- Breakfast: Pumpkin Porridge
- Lunch: Chicken and Peas Pilaf
- Dinner: Scallops with Parsnip Puree
- Snack: Oatmeal Smoothie

Tuesday
- Breakfast: Banana Yogurt Smoothie
- Lunch: Turkey and Oat Porridge
- Dinner: Cod and Asparagus Bake
- Snack: Carrot Cake

Wednesday
- Breakfast: Boiled Sweet Potatoes
- Lunch: Herbed Potato Salad
- Dinner: Oven-Poached Flounder with Stewed Green Beans
- Snack: Warm Apple Cider

Thursday
- Breakfast: Cottage Cheese with Melon
- Lunch: Turkey and Sweet Potato Hash
- Dinner: Grilled Shrimp with Green Beans Almondine
- Snack: Pear and Yogurt Smoothie

Friday
- Breakfast: Mashed Potatoes
- Lunch: Vegetable Quinoa Pilaf
- Dinner: Poached Salmon with Steamed Brussels Sprouts
- Snack: Peach Smoothie

Saturday
- Breakfast: Carrot and Ginger Juice
- Lunch: Spinach and Ricotta Stuffed Shells
- Dinner: Clam and Potato Casserole
- Snack: Vanilla and Honey Panna Cotta

Sunday
- Breakfast: Omelet with Herbs
- Lunch: Steamed Brussels Sprouts
- Dinner: Tilapia with Minted Peas
- Snack: Banana Ice Cream

Week 10

Monday
- Breakfast: Quinoa Salad
- Lunch: Chicken Porridge
- Dinner: Shrimp and Rice Pilaf
- Snack: Mango Mousse

Tuesday
- Breakfast: Soft Boiled Eggs
- Lunch: Sweet Pea and Potato Puree
- Dinner: Halibut and Zucchini
- Snack: Carrot Juice

Wednesday
- Breakfast: Barley Soup
- Lunch: Stuffed Zucchini
- Dinner: Scallop Soup
- Snack: Warm Apple Cider

Thursday
- Breakfast: Rye Bread Sandwich
- Lunch: Steamed Brussels Sprouts
- Dinner: Poached Pear and Salmon
- Snack: Vanilla and Honey Panna Cotta

Friday
- Breakfast: Basil and Spinach Smoothie
- Lunch: Herbed Turkey Steaks
- Dinner: Baked Sea Bass with Roasted Parsnips
- Snack: Pear and Yogurt Smoothie

Saturday
- Breakfast: Turkey and Sweet Potato Hash
- Lunch: Carrot and Coriander Soup
- Dinner: Oven-Poached Flounder with Stewed Green Beans
- Snack: Carrot Cake

Sunday
- Breakfast: Oatmeal Smoothie
- Lunch: Vegetable Quinoa Pilaf
- Dinner: Grilled Shrimp with Green Beans Almondine
- Snack: Banana Ice Cream

WEEKLY MEAL PLANNER + WORKBOOK

	BREAKFAST	LUNCH	DINNER	SNACKS
MONDAY				
TUESDAY				
WEDNESDAY				
THURSDAY				
FRIDAY				
SATURDAY				
SUNDAY				

Reflect on your current symptoms. How do they impact your daily life and eating habits?

....

....

....

....

....

....

WEEKLY MEAL PLANNER + WORKBOOK

	BREAKFAST	LUNCH	DINNER	SNACKS
MONDAY				
TUESDAY				
WEDNESDAY				
THURSDAY				
FRIDAY				
SATURDAY				
SUNDAY				

List three foods or beverages that you suspect might trigger discomfort or worsen your symptoms. How do you plan to avoid them?

....

....

....

....

....

WEEKLY MEAL PLANNER + WORKBOOK

	BREAKFAST	LUNCH	DINNER	SNACKS
MONDAY				
TUESDAY				
WEDNESDAY				
THURSDAY				
FRIDAY				
SATURDAY				
SUNDAY				

Consider your typical meal patterns before your ulcer diagnosis. What changes do you anticipate making to align with the stomach ulcer diet?

....

....

....

....

....

WEEKLY MEAL PLANNER + WORKBOOK

	BREAKFAST	LUNCH	DINNER	SNACKS
MONDAY				
TUESDAY				
WEDNESDAY				
THURSDAY				
FRIDAY				
SATURDAY				
SUNDAY				

Identify any dietary habits or preferences that you believe might need to change to support your healing. Why are these changes important?

....

....

....

....

....

....

WEEKLY MEAL PLANNER + WORKBOOK

	BREAKFAST	LUNCH	DINNER	SNACKS
MONDAY				
TUESDAY				
WEDNESDAY				
THURSDAY				
FRIDAY				
SATURDAY				
SUNDAY				

What are your main concerns or challenges about starting the stomach ulcer diet? How do you plan to address these concerns?

....

....

....

....

....

....

WEEKLY MEAL PLANNER + WORKBOOK

	BREAKFAST	LUNCH	DINNER	SNACKS
MONDAY				
TUESDAY				
WEDNESDAY				
THURSDAY				
FRIDAY				
SATURDAY				
SUNDAY				

List three new foods or ingredients recommended for the stomach ulcer diet that you're willing to incorporate into your meals. What benefits do you expect from including these items?

....

....

....

....

....

WEEKLY MEAL PLANNER + WORKBOOK

	BREAKFAST	LUNCH	DINNER	SNACKS
MONDAY				
TUESDAY				
WEDNESDAY				
THURSDAY				
FRIDAY				
SATURDAY				
SUNDAY				

How do you plan to navigate social situations or dining out while adhering to the stomach ulcer diet?

....

....

....

....

....

....

WEEKLY MEAL PLANNER + WORKBOOK

	BREAKFAST	LUNCH	DINNER	SNACKS
MONDAY				
TUESDAY				
WEDNESDAY				
THURSDAY				
FRIDAY				
SATURDAY				
SUNDAY				

Reflect on your current cooking skills and meal preparation routines. What adjustments might you need to make to prepare stomach ulcer diet-friendly meals?

....

....

....

....

....

....

WEEKLY MEAL PLANNER + WORKBOOK

	BREAKFAST	LUNCH	DINNER	SNACKS
MONDAY				
TUESDAY				
WEDNESDAY				
THURSDAY				
FRIDAY				
SATURDAY				
SUNDAY				

Consider your support system. How can family members or friends assist you in maintaining the stomach ulcer diet?

....

....

....

....

....

....

WEEKLY MEAL PLANNER + WORKBOOK

	BREAKFAST	LUNCH	DINNER	SNACKS
MONDAY				
TUESDAY				
WEDNESDAY				
THURSDAY				
FRIDAY				
SATURDAY				
SUNDAY				

- **What strategies will you use to track your food intake and monitor how your body responds to different foods on the stomach ulcer diet?**

....

....

....

....

....

....

WEEKLY MEAL PLANNER + WORKBOOK

	BREAKFAST	LUNCH	DINNER	SNACKS
MONDAY				
TUESDAY				
WEDNESDAY				
THURSDAY				
FRIDAY				
SATURDAY				
SUNDAY				

What are your goals for following the stomach ulcer diet? How will you measure your progress towards these goals?

....

....

....

....

....

....

WEEKLY MEAL PLANNER + WORKBOOK

	BREAKFAST	LUNCH	DINNER	SNACKS
MONDAY				
TUESDAY				
WEDNESDAY				
THURSDAY				
FRIDAY				
SATURDAY				
SUNDAY				

Reflect on any dietary restrictions or guidelines provided by your healthcare provider. How do these recommendations influence your meal planning and food choices?

....

....

....

....

....

WEEKLY MEAL PLANNER + WORKBOOK

	BREAKFAST	LUNCH	DINNER	SNACKS
MONDAY				
TUESDAY				
WEDNESDAY				
THURSDAY				
FRIDAY				
SATURDAY				
SUNDAY				

Consider any medications you're currently taking. How do you plan to coordinate your diet with your medication schedule?

....

....

....

....

....

....

Scan the QR code below to get a surprise bonus!

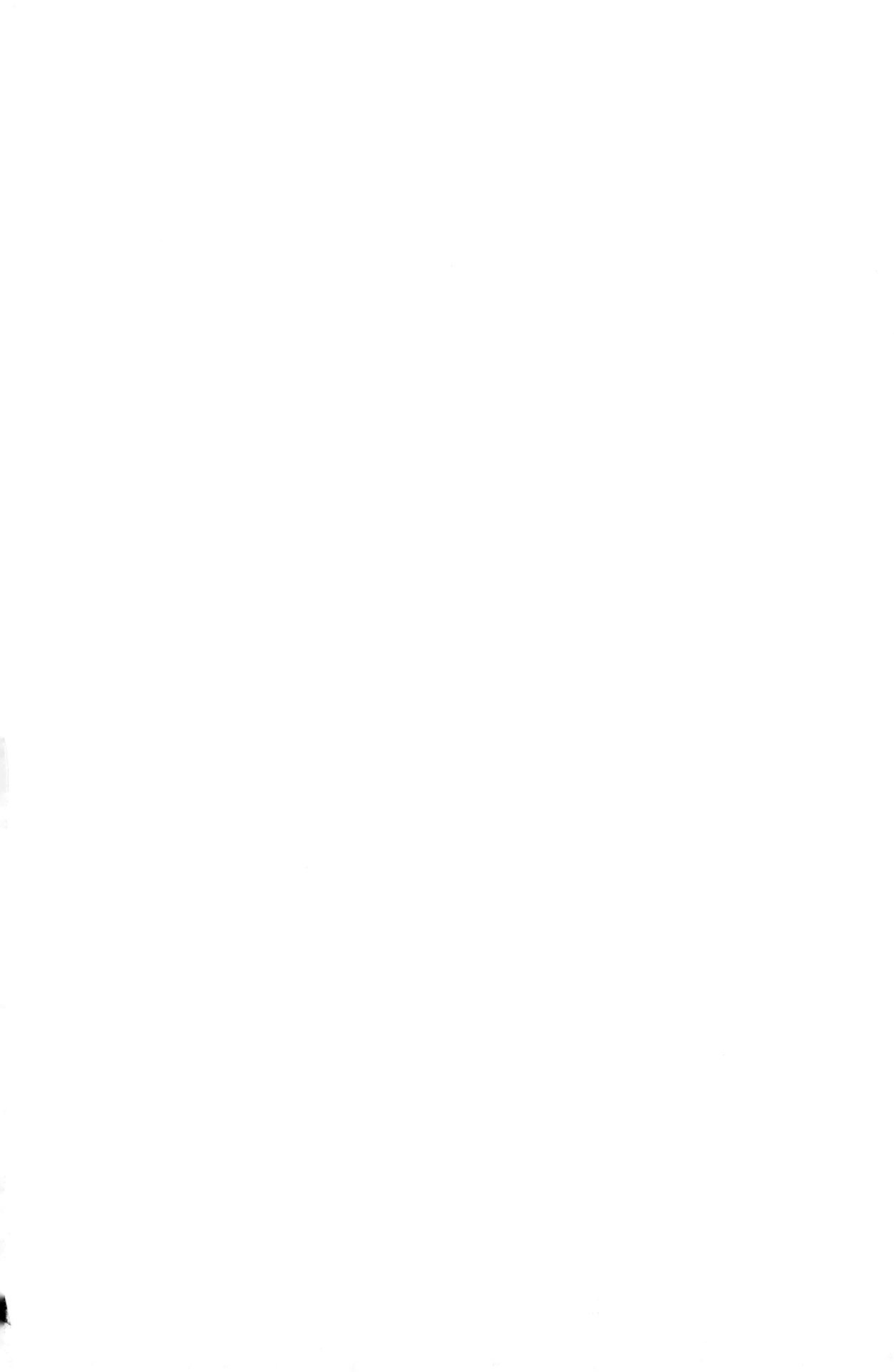

www.ingramcontent.com/pod-product-compliance
Lightning Source LLC
Chambersburg PA
CBHW082234220526
45479CB00005B/1234